This book attempts to show how important principles of genetics and evolution can be illustrated and explained using hemoglobin chemistry. The large body of information which is now available on the physical and chemical structure of the vertebrate hemoglobins, on their mode of synthesis and functioning, and on their genetic control makes such an endeavor possible. An attempt has also been made to apply some of the recent theories of molecular biology to a typical mammalian system.

Chapter 1, which is largely introductory, places hemoglobin biochemistry and hemoglobin genetics in their proper relation to other fields of human and microbial biochemical genetics. The book proceeds to treat recent findings in hemoglobin chemistry which are particularly relevant to the rest of the discussion. This is followed by a detailed examination of some recent advances in the biochem istry of abnormal inherited hemoglo normal human hemoglobins. Empha sis is on fundamental biochemica aspects rather than clinical significance. The book is based on the six Jesup Lectures presented by the author in March 1962, under the auspices of the Department of Zoology of Columbia University.

VERNON M. INGRAM is Professor of Biochemistry in the Biology Department of the Massachusetts Institute of Technology.

THE HEMOGLOBINS IN GENETICS AND EVOLUTION

Number XXII of the Columbia Biological Series

The Hemoglobins in Genetics and Evolution

VERNON M. INGRAM

COLUMBIA UNIVERSITY PRESS
New York and London
1963

Library of Congress Catalog Card Number: 63-10416
Printed in the United States of America

COLUMBIA BIOLOGICAL SERIES

Edited at Columbia University

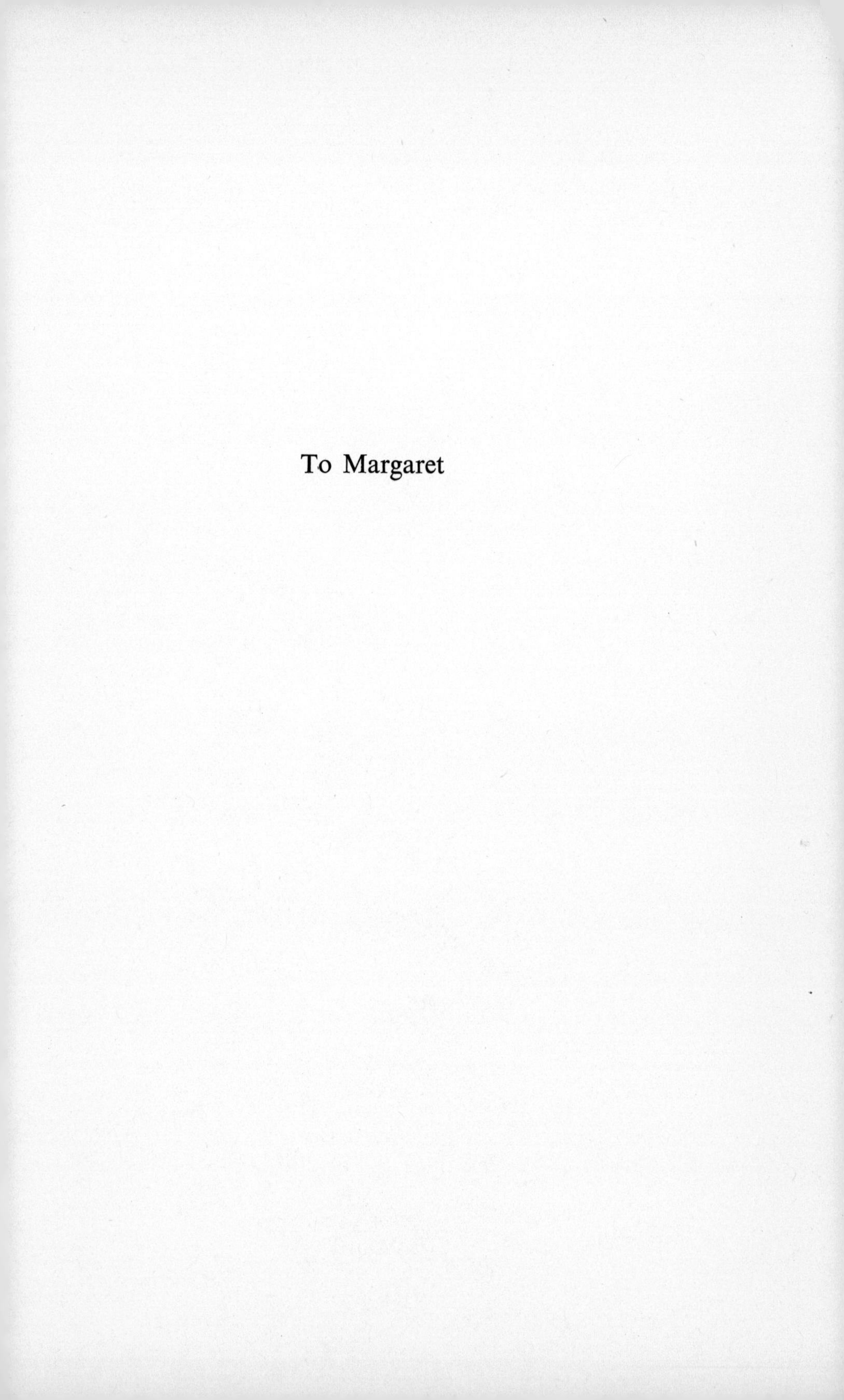

To Margaret

PREFACE

This book is based on six Jesup Lectures, delivered at Columbia University in the Department of Zoology during March, 1962. I accepted the invitation to deliver these lectures with some trepidation. The subject which I wanted to discuss is a part of such diverse areas as biochemistry, human genetics, molecular genetics, and evolution, not to mention hematology, and I felt myself to be too much of a specialist to do justice to all these aspects before an audience of biologists. In particular, an early training in classical organic chemistry and zoology followed by a gradual sliding into biochemistry and the other fields had led to the acquisition of only that knowledge which was of immediate interest and to the persistence of large areas of ignorance. Therefore, to attempt a balanced synthesis seemed too daunting. On the other hand, the temptation of the opportunity to present and develop one's own thoughts on a subject so dear to one's heart proved irresistible. The result is this book, which is offered to the reader in the hope that it will interest him and perhaps stimulate him to disagree with some of the ideas put forward.

In such a short book, it has been impossible to include reference to everyone whose work would have been relevant. A rather arbitrary choice was often necessary, with apologies to those who have had to be omitted, but not through lack of an appreciation of their work.

VERNON M. INGRAM

Cambridge, Mass.
July, 1962

ACKNOWLEDGMENTS

In the first instance, I would like to thank most sincerely Dr. Howard Levene and the committee who organize the Jesup Lectures for their kind invitation. My visits to the Department of Zoology and Botany during that period were made most pleasant and interesting through the kindness of my hosts, particularly Drs. Dunn, Moore, Ryan, Sager, and Taylor, as well as many others.

Much of the original work reported here was done either by, or in collaboration with, Drs. Baglioni, Hunt, and Stretton. In particular, I would like to acknowledge the help and stimulation of many critical discussions with Dr. Baglioni and Dr. Stretton concerning some of the more theoretical ideas put forward here, without, however, wishing to evade my responsibility for them.

Many authors and publishers have been most generous in allowing me to reproduce certain drawings and photographs. Proper acknowledgment is made to them in the appropriate places. I am grateful to the staff of the Columbia University Press for their help, efficiency, and patience.

Finally, I would like to thank my secretary, Miss Barbara Garrelts, without whose help this book would not exist.

V. M. I.

CONTENTS

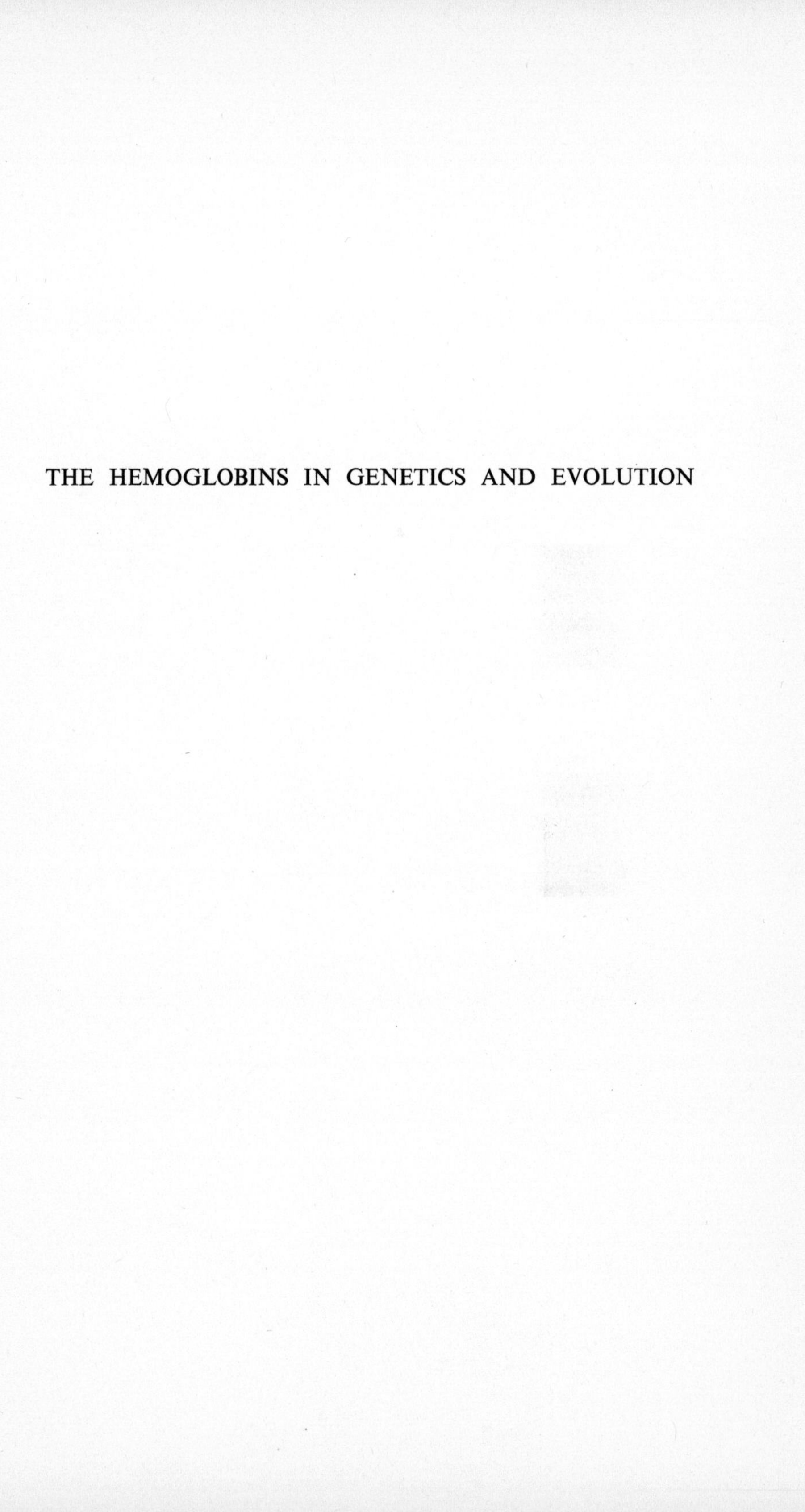

THE HEMOGLOBINS IN GENETICS AND EVOLUTION

1

INTRODUCTION

The six lectures transcribed in this book were designed to present a personal view of biochemical genetics and evolution. These two topics were treated almost entirely in terms of the biochemistry of the hemoglobins and no attempt was made to give a balanced view of these large areas of scientific endeavor. The same plan was followed when the pleasant task of giving the Jesup lectures (March, 1962) in the congenial environment of the Zoology Department of Columbia University turned into the more arduous job of putting one's thoughts and prejudices onto paper. Not even the more restricted field of the hemoglobins, normal and abnormal, will be extensively reviewed here, since this has been adequately done in several very recent reviews (see later). Only some aspects of particular interest to the author will be discussed.

Most books that are concerned with biochemical genetics open with a reference to Garrod's work early in this century. This is as it should be, since it was he who in 1902 described the first human biochemical inherited disease, alkaptonuria, and who coined the term "inborn errors of metabolism" (see Garrod, 1923). This name, which has persisted as a most useful description of these diseases, underlines the point that we are dealing here with an inherited defect on the biochemical level. In alkaptonuria one can actually point to the defect as the absence of the active enzyme which normally converts homogentisic acid to maleylacetoacetic acid as part of the metabolism of tyrosine. More recently, the term "inborn error of metabolism" has come to mean an "error" or an alteration in the chemical structure of a biochemically important substance. In this last sense, we may talk of the inherited hemoglobinopathies as "inborn errors of metabolism" of a kind which allows us to study the basic defect directly, in spite of the fact that a hemoglobin defect is a metabolic defect only in the widest sense of the word.

A second important step in the development of this subject came in 1949 when Pauling coined the term "molecular disease." In that year, Pauling, Itano, Singer, and Wells (1949) discovered that patients with sickle-cell anemia carried a hemoglobin which was electrophoretically different from normal hemoglobin. It seemed likely even then, that such a difference was due to a definite biochemical abnormality at the molecular level. Also in 1949 came the demonstration by Neel and also by Beet, that this "inborn error," this "molecular disease," was inherited as a simple Mendelian factor, with the heterozygote possessing the hemoglobins characteristic of both the normal and the mutant alleles.

These are the most important landmarks for the development of the story of the human hemoglobin abnormalities. Since then there has been a very great deal of research in this area, so that we now have a reasonably coherent picture of the biochemical genetics of this protein. Much of this work has been summarized in several recent reviews (Itano, 1957; Lehmann and Ager, 1960; Rucknagel and Neel, 1961; Baglioni, 1962).

A third milestone was the formulation of the "one gene-one enzyme" hypothesis by Beadle and Tatum (1941) which is fundamental to that part of our picture which deals with genetic control of the structure of any particular protein.

GENETIC CONTROL OF CELLULAR ACTIVITIES

It is a commonplace nowadays in molecular biology to state the relationship between a gene and its product as the relationship between genetic DNA which makes template RNA which in turn makes protein (Figure 1-1). The one gene-one enzyme hypothesis leads to the proposition that the chemical structure of the relevant portion of DNA will produce a definite chemical structure in a protein. It is this relationship and its ramifications which we will examine in this book, taking our examples largely from the biochemical work on the hemoglobins. Just as a normal gene will produce, in this view, a normal protein molecule, so the effects of a gene mutation are felt as a chemical alteration in the structure of that protein, provided that this protein is the first protein product of the gene. One can well imagine that some proteins are one step further removed from the gene than are for example the peptide chains of hemoglobin. Some proteins have carbohydrate constituents

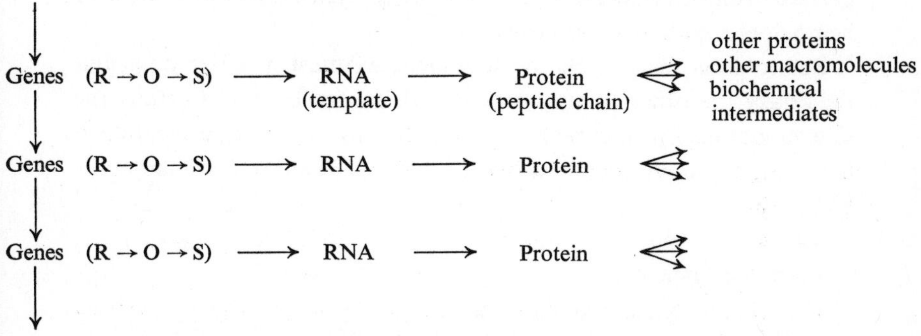

FIGURE 1-1. Scheme of the genetic control of protein synthesis
Three successive generations are shown. R: regulator gene; O: operator gene; S: structural gene. (See Jacob and Monod, 1961.)

attached to them, put there by the action of some enzymes. These enzymes are themselves proteins and are made by their own genes. A mutation in one of these genes may alter or delete the function of such an enzyme and may ultimately show up as an alteration in the carbohydrate portions of one or more other proteins, leaving their peptide chain sequences perfectly normal. This would be a less direct effect of a gene mutation on protein structure.

The complex system of genetic control (Figure 1-1) leaves of course a great deal unsaid, particularly in terms of the relationship between the types of gene (regulator, operator, structural) or indeed the need to postulate them in a mammalian system. Nevertheless, the scheme provides a convenient and useful way for examining the findings of biochemical genetics and for directing the planning of experiments.

This scheme of cellular control is supposed to be applicable in bacteria as well as in mammals. In fact the best studied examples for the correspondence between genetic and protein structure come from the bacterial systems (Dreyer, 1960; Jacob and Monod, 1961; Garen, Levinthal, and Rothman, 1961; Helinski and Yanofsky, 1962). The same is true for the demonstration of the role of template (messenger) RNA (see for example Brenner *et al.*, 1961; Gros *et al.*, 1961). However, we will confine ourselves in this book to applying the principles derived from the more tractable microbial systems to the control of hemoglobin synthesis and structure.

Before proceeding to the hemoglobins, we must however point out that there are other human proteins which can be used to study the scheme outlined in Figure 1-1, of which only two will be mentioned here, glucose-6-phosphate dehydrogenase (G-6-P-D) and haptoglobin.

G-6-P-D DEFICIENCY

The inherited glucose-6-phosphate dehydrogenase deficiency has been demonstrated in many Negroes (10 percent) in this country who have a severe hemolytic anemia when certain drugs are administered (see Marks, 1960; also Marks *et al.*, 1961; Ramot *et al.*, 1961; Adinolfi *et al.*, 1961). These drugs include sulfanilamide and primaquine. The usual form of the condition is inherited as a sex-linked gene of intermediate dominance. The biochemical reaction which seems to be involved in this disease and which is mediated by the enzyme G-6-P-D is the following: glucose-6-phosphate + 2 TPN → 6-phosphogluconic acid + 2 $TPNH^+$. The TPNH which is produced is used in many ways in the cell; for example it is used to keep glutathione reduced.

Siniscalco, Bernini, and Latte (1961) found that in Sardinia G-6-P-D deficiency is linked to color blindness and to hemophilia. There is still some controversy as to whether this disease is really all of one kind in different parts of the world. Although the clinical symptons are similar, this is probably a group of different enzyme defects. Another way in which this deficiency is detected in Italy and elsewhere is after ingestion of the fava bean which in persons with this deficiency will also cause a hemolytic anemia. Siniscalco *et al.* (1961) found that G-6-P-D deficiency is strongly correlated in portions of Sardinia with the presence, either today or in the past, of malaria. This is an example of balanced polymorphism, where the disadvantage of a gene is balanced by some selective advantage of the heterozygote (usually), leading to an unexpectedly high level of frequency of a deleterious gene. We will come across other examples of this phenomenon in the hemoglobin system. After all, the possession of G-6-P-D deficiency is deleterious—nobody knows how deleterious exactly and yet the frequency is high. Since there is a positive statistical correlation between the distribution of malaria and the distribution of this gene, one is tempted to postulate that partial protection against malaria is the mechanism. There is as yet no actual evidence for such protection in this particular biochemical abnormality. When we turn to sickle cell anemia later, we will find that there is a similar situation of balanced polymorphism, but there is now considerable evidence that malaria really is involved in increasing the frequency of the sickle cell anemia gene. In the case of the G-6-P-D deficiency we have only a correlation at the moment. Sardinia is a favorable place for studying balanced polymorphism, because there are villages high up in the mountains with little malaria and other villages in the lowlands, where there is, or was, a lot of malaria. And just as G-6-P-D deficiency is positively correlated with malaria, so it is negatively correlated with altitude.

The kind of G-6-P-D deficiency which Ramot *et al.* (1961) have studied in Israel amongst the Jews may not be the same condition. She also found that G-6-P-D deficiency is linked to color blindness, but this time the genes are in repulsion, whereas in Sardinia they were in coupling. Ramot also studied the level of the enzymes in tissues other than the red cell (Table 1-1) and found different levels of enzyme activity in affected individuals, indicating that the gene mutation affects the enzyme in a variety of cell types, if not in all.

It is not always clear that the same structural gene is involved in making enzymes of similar function in different tissues. There is some chemical evidence that the enzyme lysozyme in the spleen and the brain of dogs is different chemically; maybe there are different, though related, structural genes involved in producing these enzymes. On the other hand, as far as human G-6-P-D is concerned, it looks as if only

TABLE 1-1

G6PD ACTIVITY IN VARIOUS TISSUES

Tissue	*Number*	*Control*	*Number*	*"Mutants"*
Erythrocytes°	103	12.6 ± 1.18	55	1.08 ± 1.04
Platelets°°	56	0.127 ± 0.038	34	0.024 ± 0.017
Leucocytes°°	26	34.70 ± 11.20	25	7.59 ± 2.72
Saliva**	26	8.00 ± 6.3	14	0.54 ± 0.4
Liver*	18	0.112 ± 0.038	3	0.010–0.030
Skin**	9	2.6–20.9	2	0.167–1.6

° Units = ΔOD/g Hb/min. ± standard deviation.
°° Units = ΔOD/10^9 cells/min.
** Units = ΔOD/mg protein/min.
* Units = ΔOD/100 mg wet Liver Tissue/min.

one structural gene is involved; the mutation, whatever it is, affects the G-6-P-D enzyme similarly in the various tissues. Marks *et al.* (1961, 1962) have reported studies of the biochemical properties of the G-6-P-D enzymes taken from normal individuals and from a variety of mutants, which demonstrate that chemically different enzymes may be found (Table 1-2). For example, in the normal subject and in the affected Negro subject the enzyme has a certain mobility in starch gel electrophoresis; but in one Italian family, the electrophoretic mobility of the G-6-P-D enzyme was increased 35 percent; therefore we would suspect that a different protein is made in these individuals, pointing to at least two types of G-6-P-D deficiency.

In the hemoglobins we are very fortunate because the protein is easy to prepare. Even the mutant hemoglobins are usually easy to obtain. We can therefore settle more easily the question whether we are dealing with a mutant protein or with different rates of production in the hemoglobin abnormalities.

THE HAPTOGLOBINS

Another example of an inherited abnormality in the human system is the haptoglobins. These human proteins maybe a type of antibody, at least they combine specifically with hemoglobin (Jayle and Boussier, 1955; Moretti *et al.*, 1957). It looks as if one molecule of haptoglobin

TABLE 1-2

PROPERTIES OF GLUCOSE-6-P DEHYDROGENASE PURIFIED FROM RED CELLS OF NORMAL SUBJECTS AND PERSONS WITH A DEFICIENCY IN THIS ENZYME

Source	*RBC enzyme activity*	K_{m1} *TPN*	K_m *G6P*	K_m *2-D-G6P*	K_m *nicotin-amide*	*pH optima*	*Electro-phoresis*
	Units/gmHgb	$M \times 10^{-6}$	$M \times 10^{-5}$	$M \times 10^{-3}$	$M \times 10^{-2}$		*Percent*
Normal subjects (7)	11.5–18.2	3.4–7.1	3.5–5.6	3.0–3.6	2.0	8.5–9.3	100.0
Affected subjects:							
Negro males (4)	1.2–4.1	4.4–8.0	3.7–4.1	4.2–5.0	2.0–3.0	8.5–9.3	100.0
Negro female (1)	8.7	3.6	4.0	4.0	2.0	8.5–9.3	100.0
Barbieri males (2)	6.5–7.2	12–28	5.6–8.0	2.5–5.9	2.0	8.5–9.3	135.0
Barbieri females (1)	8.0	24	6.6	5.0	2.0	8.5–9.3	131.0
Caucasian male (1)	0.9	9.2	3.4–6.7	4.5	—	8.5–9.3	100.0
Caucasian female (1)	0.8	5.0	2.8	—	—	8.5–9.3	100.0
Caucasian-Negro male (1)	1.5	14	7.5	7.2	—	8.6–9.3	—

Abbreviations: TPN, triphosphopyridine nucleotide; G6P, glucose-6 phosphate; 2-D-G6P, 2-desoxy-glucose-6-phosphate. Values indicated in table are range of values where more than one enzyme preparation was studied.

will combine with one molecule of hemoglobin, that is, each haptoglobin molecule has one combining site. This may only be true for the so-called type 1-1 haptoglobin (Smithies and Connell, 1959); type 2-1 or 2-2 may combine with more than one hemoglobin molecule for reasons which will be apparent later. Usually a typical antibody has two combining sites; thereby it is able to form a three-dimensional network with the protein with which it reacts and to precipitate that protein. Haptoglobin does not precipitate hemoglobin, but it does form a strong complex which seems to be a mechanism for removing free hemoglobin from solution in the serum. During a hemolytic crisis, hemoglobin is liberated into serum, the haptoglobin combines with it and the haptoglobin-hemoglobin complex is then eliminated. After a severe hemolytic crisis one does not find any haptoglobin, because it has been used up. There are actually many people who have no haptoglobin at any time; about three or four percent of some of the Negro populations in Africa show this absence of haptoglobin (Allison *et al.*, 1958). This lack of haptoglobin does not seem to be disadvantageous, so that perhaps the haptoglobin is not an essential part of the biochemical mechanism of the body. On the other hand, there may be other functions of this protein of which we know nothing yet.

Smithies, in 1956, introduced a beautiful technique for the separation of serum proteins (reviewed in Smithies, 1959). He performed electrophoresis of these proteins in starch gel, which gives a much better separation and characterization of human proteins than had been possible before. This technique enabled him to see these haptoglobins; on screening populations he discovered that there were three distinct types of individuals with respect to their haptoglobins (Smithies and Connell, 1959). These were called types 1-1, 2-1, and 2-2. The type 1-1 was from a homozygote Hp^1/Hp^1, the 2-2 was the other homozygote (Hp^2/Hp^2) of the allelic system and the 2-1 type was produced by the heterozygote Hp^1/Hp^2. The molecular weight of type 1-1 haptoglobin is about 85,000 (Moretti *et al.*, 1957); it is not entirely a simple protein, but also contains some carbohydrate, which was shown by Jayle and Boussier (1955) some time before Smithies' work. Parker and Bearn (1962) have found recently that neuraminidase, which presumably removes a carbohydrate constituent, alters the electrophoretic mobility of human haptoglobin 1-1.

Figure 1-2 shows a starch gel electrophoresis taken from Smithies' work, illustrating on the left the three types of haptoglobins which are found. The homozygote, Hp^2/Hp^2, produces a series of bands, some stronger and some weaker, probably due to association of this type of molecule. The heterozygote produces a series of proteins *intermediate* in nature between the two homozygotes. Reduced type 1-1 and 2-2 show single protein bands in different electrophoretic positions. The heterozygote, 2-1, after reduction, has both the bands characteristic of 1-1 and of 2-2. The reduced proteins show phenotypes which correspond to the alleles in the genotypes.

In the abnormal hemoglobins, the heterozygote shows both forms of hemoglobin molecules of the allelic system *without* any previous degradation of the protein. One does not get truly hybrid molecules made up of peptide chains produced by the two allelic genes, as happens in the haptoglobins. This is a very clear distinction between the two systems.

One can recognize two types of peptide chains in the haptoglobins: α chains and β chains. Figure 1-2 shows only the α chains, since in this system of electrophoresis the β chains remain insoluble at the origin. But recently it has been possible (Connell, Dixon, and Smithies, 1962) to move the β chain away from the origin and to show that they are the same in these three types. The mutational differences which distinguish the haptoglobin types reside in the α chain.

It appears that in fact there are three kinds of type 1-1 haptoglobin, the socalled 1^{Fast}-1^{Fast}, 1^{Fast}-1^{Slow} and 1^{Slow}-1^{Slow}, referring to the speed of their α chain components in electrophoresis (Connell, Dixon, and Smithies, 1962).

Figure 1-3 illustrates in schematic form some of the chemical findings of Smithies, Connell, and Dixon (1962), derived from digestion of the peptide chains with chymotrypsin and from isolation and fingerprinting of the fragments in a way similar to the methods discussed in chapter 3. Smithies has shown that the Hp^2 peptide chain differs from $Hp1^{\text{Fast}}$ and $Hp1^{\text{Slow}}$ α peptide chains by being almost twice as long. By careful

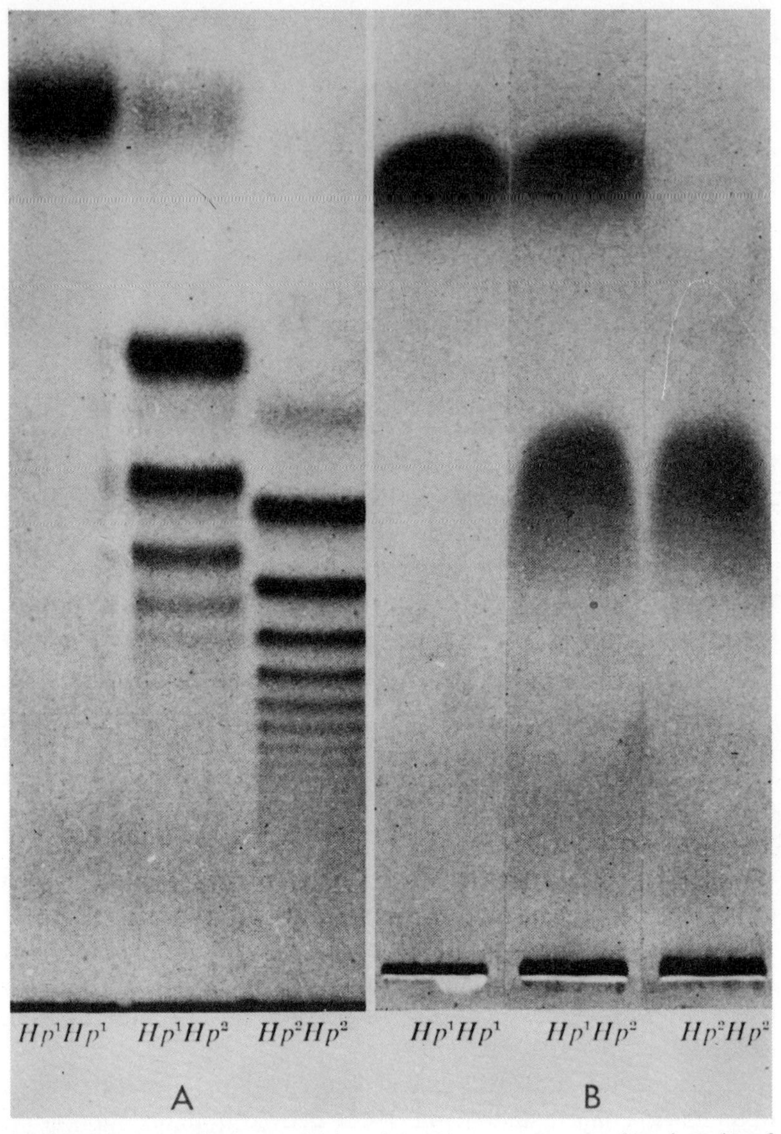

FIGURE 1-2. The haptoglobins of the three genotypes Hp^1/Hp^1, Hp^1/Hp^2, Hp^2/Hp^2

A: purified haptoglobins, B: haptoglobins after reduction of disulfide bonds and alkylation of the liberated —SH groups. Electrophoresis in starch gel, pH 3.2. By permission of Dr. Oliver Smithies.

purification and fingerprinting of enzymatic digests of these chains he deduced (Smithies, Connell, and Dixon, 1962) that most of the peptides derived from the Hp^1 chain are represented in the Hp^2 chain, but that the Hp^2 chains seem to be composed of one $Hp1^{Fast}$ chain and one

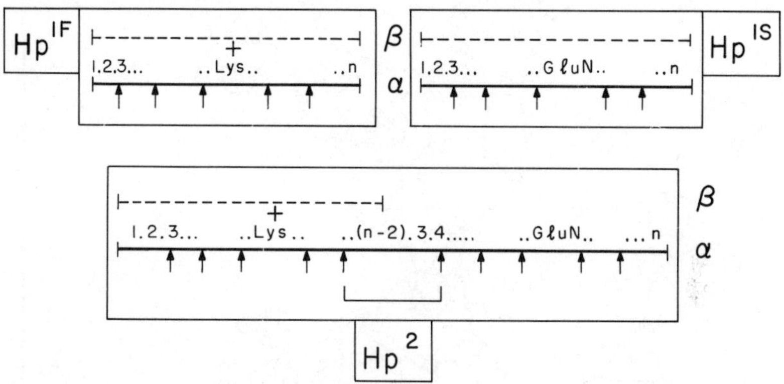

FIGURE 1-3. Schematic representation of the chemical differences in the α peptide chains of haptoglobins Hp^{1F} (= 1^{Fast}), Hp^{1S} (= 1^{Slow}) and Hp^2 (Based on the results of Smithies *et al.*, 1962.)

$Hp1^{Slow}$ chain joined together with a few amino acids missing at the junction. $Hp1^{Fast}$ differs from $Hp1^{Slow}$ by having a lysine residue instead of a glutamic acid or glutamine residue (see Figure 1-3), thus accounting for the electrophoretic differences. The pronounced difference in electrophoresis between the whole molecules of Hp^1 and Hp^2 is due to the

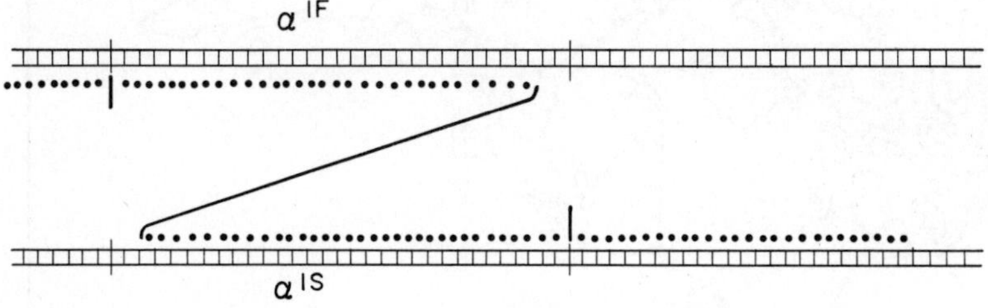

FIGURE 1-4. Schematic representation of an unequal crossing over mechanism to explain the origin of the α^2 chain of Hp^2 from a heterozygote Hp^{1F}/Hp^{1S} which has an α^{1F} and an α^{1S} gene

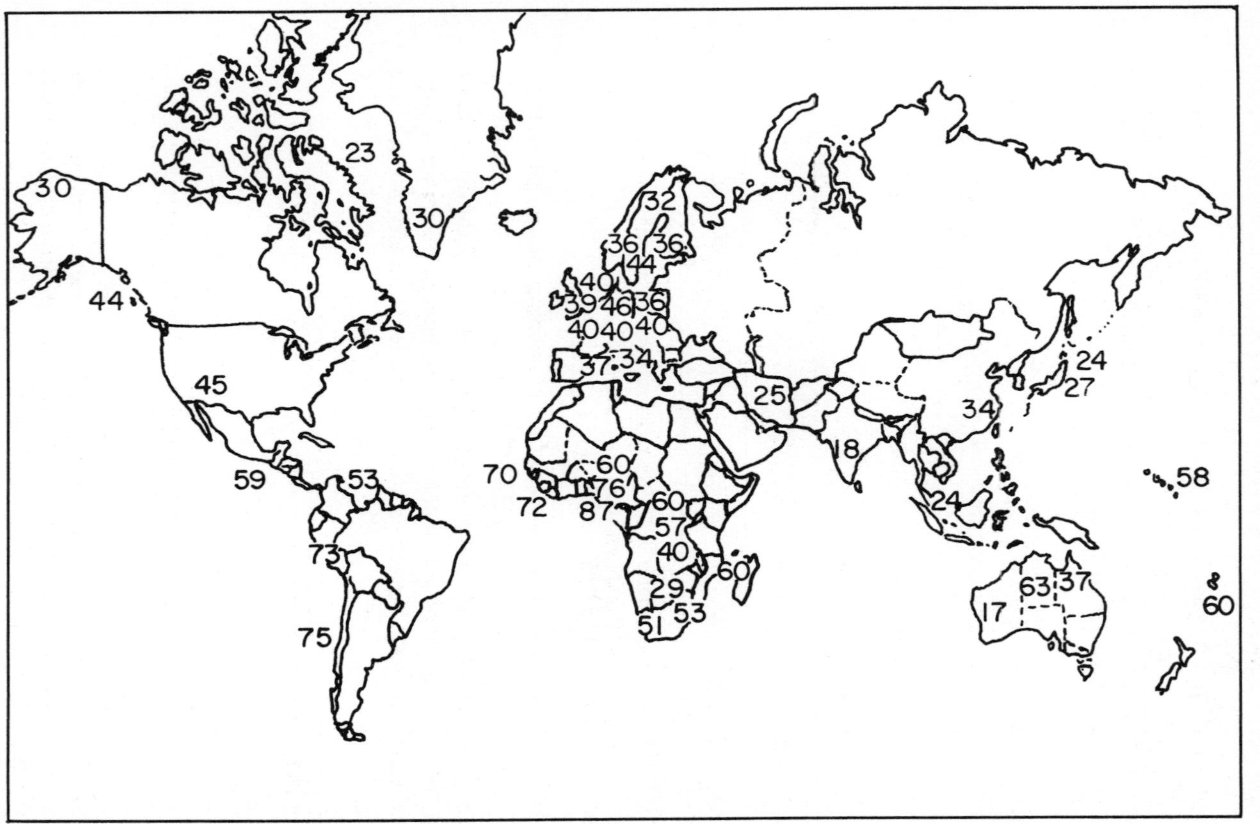

FIGURE 1-5. Polymorphism of human haptoglobin
Gene frequency (percent) of the haptoglobin—1 allele (alleles). (Parker and Bearn, 1961.)

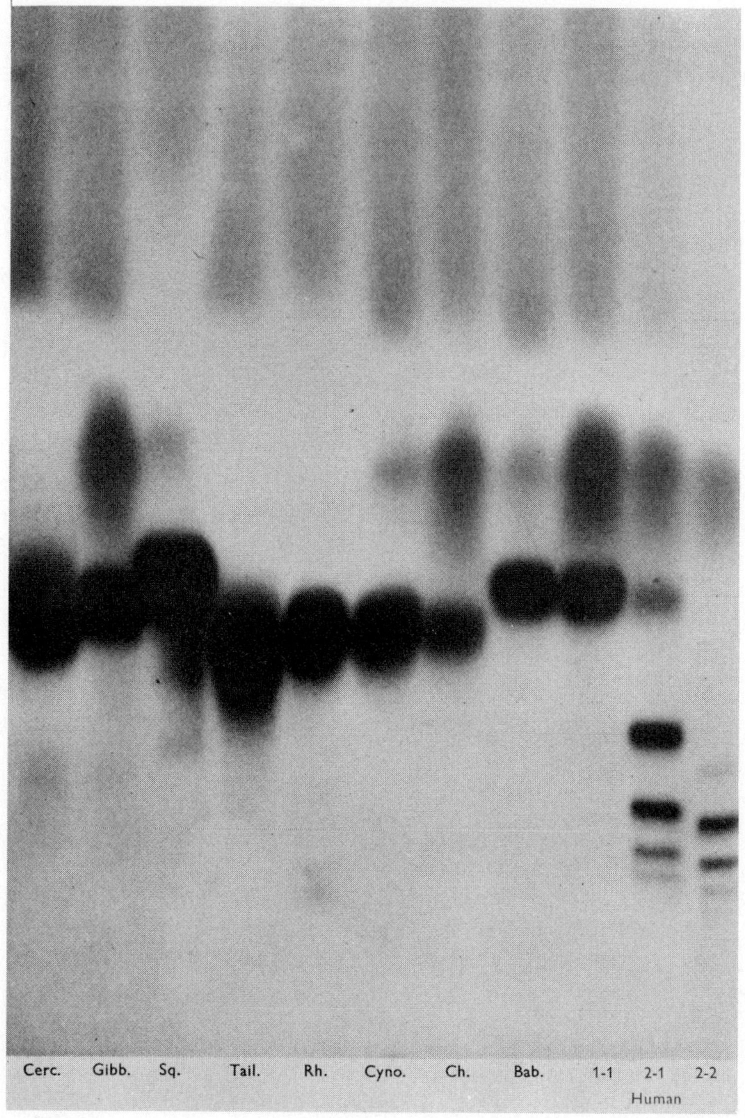

FIGURE 1-6. Haptoglobin variation in humans and primates; benzidine stain after vertical starch gel electrophoresis

Serum samples from left are from the cercopithecus monkey, gibbon, squirrel monkey, tailless macaque, rhesus monkey, cynomolgus monkey, chimpanzee, baboon and the three common human phenotypes. In several samples an excess hemoglobin band is seen slightly ahead of the human Hp 1–1 band: hemoglobin is also seen bound to albumin. (Parker and Bearn, 1961.)

great increase in complexity of the molecule. It is interesting that the gene controlling the Hp^2 α chain must have arisen from a heterozygote carrying both the $Hp1^{Fast}$ and the $Hp1^{Slow}$ gene, since both the amino acid substitutions characteristic of these two chains are present in the Hp^2 α chain. Presumably this Hp^2 α gene might have arisen (Figure 1-4) by nonhomologous crossing over operating in the $Hp1^{Fast}/Hp1^{Slow}$ heterozygote. Such an event could lead not to a clean gene duplication, but rather to an incomplete gene duplication, resulting in a single gene of almost twice the usual length, but nevertheless operating as a single gene.

In studies of the distribution of the haptoglobin types (Parker and Bearn, 1961), it has been shown that the Hp^2 gene is in fact found with high frequencies in many parts of the world, particularly in India where it is the predominant form (Figure 1-5). Now as we have seen, the gene controlling the Hp^2 α chains must have arisen subsequent to the existence of the $Hp1^{Fast}$ and $Hp1^{Slow}$ genes, since it contains elements of both. Presumably the Hp^2 gene confers a selective advantage, particularly in India, on the person possessing it to such an extent that since it arose it has begun to displace the older Hp^1 genes. We have here an example of evolution in action. Presumably the spread of the Hp^2 gene is not yet complete; whether it will ever be complete is of course not known. Just what this selective advantage is, is also not clear, although one might postulate that the doubling in size and the consequent ability of the molecule to polymerize, might lead to a more efficient function in its combination with hemoglobin, if indeed that is its function.

The argument for the recent evolution of the type 2-2 haptoglobin is strengthened by Parker and Bearn's finding (1961) that eight other primates had a haptoglobin pattern similar to the human type 1-1, i.e., a single component (Figure 1-6). The multiple bands characteristic of Hp^2 gene may well be a feature peculiar to humans.

2

THE STRUCTURE AND SYNTHESIS OF HEMOGLOBIN

Everybody who has worked with hemoglobin has been helped enormously by the fact that this protein has been under intensive study by chemists, physical chemists, and biochemists for a long time. This fortunate circumstance has made it possible to interpret the clinical findings on genetically altered hemoglobins very much more easily than if one had had to start with a protein about which little was known. In order to discuss the abnormal hemoglobins we will in this chapter consider some aspects of the structural chemistry of hemoglobin and also some aspects of the biosynthesis of this protein.

First of all it will be necessary to define a few terms concerning protein structure (Low and Edsall, 1956). By the *primary* structure of a protein we understand the covalent structure of the polypeptide chains and in particular the sequence of the amino acids; by *secondary* structure we understand the regular arrangement in space of such polypeptide chains as for example in the α helix of Corey, Pauling and Branson (1951); the *tertiary* structure is the arrangement of such helices in space giving the super folding of the molecule; finally, the *quarternary* structure of the protein is the assembly of subunits composed of the individual polypeptide chains to form the final molecule.

Hemoglobin has four such subunits (Schroeder, 1959): two α polypeptide chains and two β polypeptide chains, each arranged as a more or less spherical subunit (Perutz *et al.*, 1960). The complete hemoglobin molecule, the tetramer, has a molecular weight of around 67,000. It seems likely that most vertebrate hemoglobins are made up in this way, with the exception of the hemoglobins from cyclostomes. Hemoglobin is considered to be a compound protein in the sense that it is composed of the protein globin and of four heme groups; these are molecules composed of protoporphyrin rings each containing at the center an iron atom. Each of the four subunits contains therefore one peptide chain together with its heme group. It is the iron atom (Fe^{++}) at the center of each heme group which is functionally the most important part of the molecule, since it is here that oxygen molecules attach themselves reversably during the oxygenation and deoxygenation of hemoglobin in its normal physiological role.

THE HEMOGLOBIN TYPES

The normal adult human hemoglobin (hemoglobin A or Hb A) is often written as $\alpha_2^A\beta_2^A$ (Figure 2-1) to show that it is composed of two

Adult	$\alpha_2^A \; \beta_2^A$
Fetal	$\alpha_2^A \; \gamma_2^F$
A2	$\alpha_2^A \; \delta_2^{A2}$
Hemoglobin H	β_4^A
Hemoglobin "Barts"	γ_4^F

FIGURE 2-1. The different types of human hemoglobins
Included are two examples of abnormal hemoglobins which are peculiar in having four identical subunits; they are discussed in chapters 3 and 4.

α peptide chains and two β peptide chains. The superscript A shows that the molecule is of the genetically normal, adult type. The human fetus on the other hand has a different type of hemoglobin (reviewed in White and Beaven, 1959) which can be readily distinguished chemically, but which has the same overall molecular complexity. Human fetal hemoglobin is composed of four peptide chains: two α polypeptide chains, the same as in the adult type, and two γ polypeptide chains chemically distinguishable from the β polypeptide chains (Schroeder and Matsuda, 1958). We see then that half the molecule is identical with the adult type, but that the other half is different.

Also, the normal human adult has a minor hemoglobin component (Kunkel and Wallenius, 1955), called hemoglobin A_2, which is electrophoretically distinguishable from the others. Hemoglobin A_2 also has four polypeptide chains in its molecule, two α chains, which are identical with those in the adult protein and in fetal hemoglobin, and in addition two δ peptide chains (Ingram and Stretton, 1961). The symbol δ is used to indicate that these peptide chains are distinguishable in their primary structure from the β and γ peptide chains and are also under separate genetic control (see chapter 4). Altogether then, there are four types of polypeptide chain which make up the three types of hemoglobin found in the human (Figure 2-1)—the α, β, γ, and δ chains. There is very good genetic evidence to indicate that these four types of peptide chain have their primary structure controlled by four different structural genes. We will discuss the genetic evidence for this statement in a later chapter.

The hemoglobins of vertebrates are strikingly similar in their overall structure, with the notable exception of the hemoglobins found in certain cyclostomata (see in Gratzer and Allison, 1960). The vertebrate hemoglobins are all composed of four polypeptide chains of two kinds; for these we can write as in the human a formula of the type of $\alpha_2\beta_2$. In addition there is evidence now that multiple forms of hemoglobin are to be found in certain mammals. An excellent review of this subject has recently been published by Gratzer & Allison (1960). In spite of the overall similarity there are of course structural differences between, for example, rabbit hemoglobin and human hemoglobin. These are differences in the amino acid sequences, but they are really quite few in number and the overall resemblance of the molecule is striking (Muller, 1961; Diamond and Braunitzer, 1962; Naughton and Dintzis, 1962).

Two other types of human hemoglobin are illustrated in Figure 2-1; these are hemoglobin H (Rigas *et al.*, 1955; Gouttas *et al.*, 1955;

Jones *et al.*, 1959) and hemoglobin Barts (Fessas and Papaspyrou, 1957; Ager and Lehmann, 1958; Hunt and Lehmann, 1959) composed respectively of four β peptide chains and four γ peptide chains. Both are to be classified as abnormal hemoglobins, because they are produced in certain conditions of inherited hemolytic anemia. There seems to be a relative overproduction of β or γ peptide chains within a cell leading to tetramer formation of the type illustrated in Figure 2-1. The conditions under which hemoglobin H and Barts can be found will be discussed later.

One of the characteristic features of the hemoglobin molecule is its high degree of symmetry. The molecule can be divided into two identical halves, each containing one α and one β peptide chain. The two halves are related by a dyad axis of symmetry. It follows that any structural feature of an α peptide chains, for example, is faithfully reproduced in the other α peptide chain of the molecule. Later, when we discuss the mutational alterations of hemoglobin, we will find that in every case a particular amino acid alteration is to be found in both α peptide chains or, as the case may be, in both β peptide chains of a molecule. The chemical work necessary for pinpointing mutational alterations in the primary structure of the abnormal hemoglobins is therefore reduced to half.

X-RAY STRUCTURE OF HEMOGLOBIN

The secondary, tertiary, and quarternary structure of hemoglobin has been worked out in considerable detail by Perutz and his colleagues in England (1960–62). Although the hemoglobin with which he worked is horse hemoglobin, there are good reasons for thinking that human hemoglobin is quite similar in its overall structure. The pictures reproduced here (Figures 2-2 and 2-3, 2-3a, 2-3b) are those of horse hemoglobin. The models which are shown are the result of x-ray studies on single crystals of this hemoglobin. At present this model is at low resolution (5.5A) which means that it is not yet possible to see the outlines of individual atoms or even of groups of atoms such as the amino acids. On the other hand it is easily possible to see the coiling of the peptide chains, as well as the overall architecture of the individual subunits and of the complete molecule. This gives us a most important view of the relation between the primary structure and the ultimate molecule. In Figure 2-2 we see a hemoglobin molecule dissected into two asymmetrical half molecules composed of either two α chains

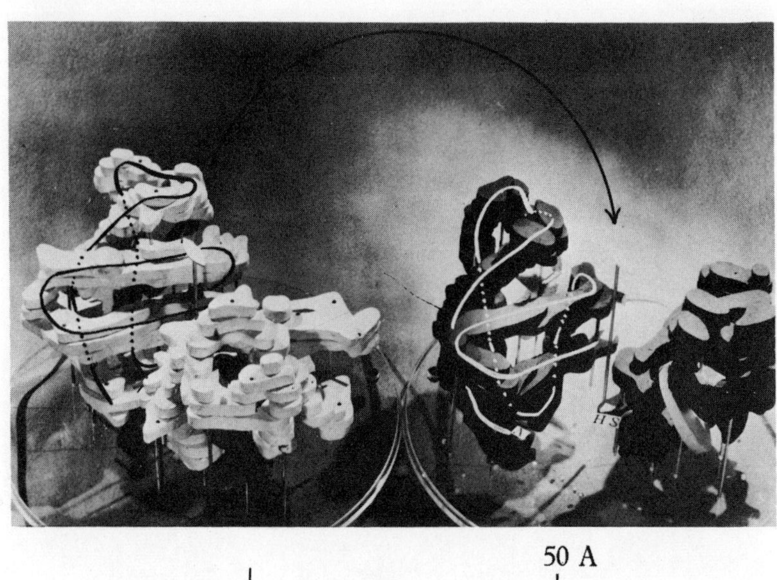

FIGURE 2-2. Model of horse hemoglobin at 5.5 A resolution
The two inner subunits (α_2-white, β_2-black) have been separated to show how they will fit together. The N-terminus of some chains, the heme groups, and the general coiling of the chains can be seen. The reactive sulfhydryl (—SH) group of the β chain is visible in one of the β chains. From a photograph kindly supplied by Dr. M. F. Perutz.

(white) or two β chains (black). It is very striking that the overall folding of α and β peptide chains resemble one another, but are not quite identical. This close similarity reflects the great resemblance between the amino acid sequences of these two types of chain (Figure 2-5). The fact that there are also differences in the amino acid sequences is reflected in the fact that the coiling of α and β peptide chains is not quite identical.

By somewhat similar x-ray methods Kendrew and coworkers (1960, 1961) have been able to study the related protein myoglobin. This protein is only a quarter of the size of hemoglobin, consisting of a

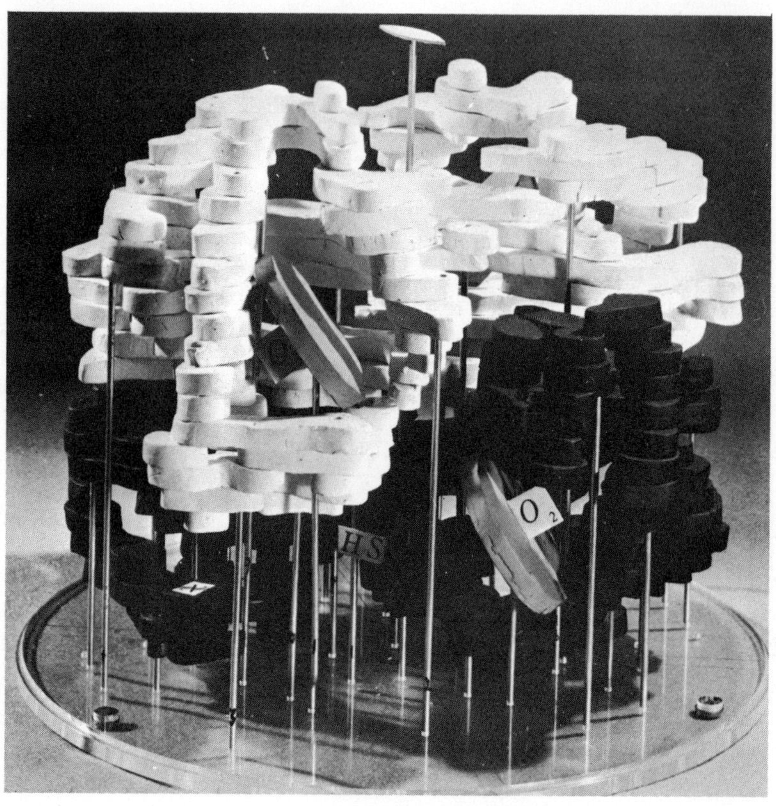

FIGURE 2-3. Model of horse hemoglobin at 5.5 A resolution From a photograph kindly supplied by Dr. M. F. Perutz.

single polypeptide chain and a single heme group. It is found in muscle where it combines reversibly with oxygen and acts as a store for oxygen. Kendrew has been able to show a striking resemblance in the architecture of myoglobin and individual hemoglobin peptide

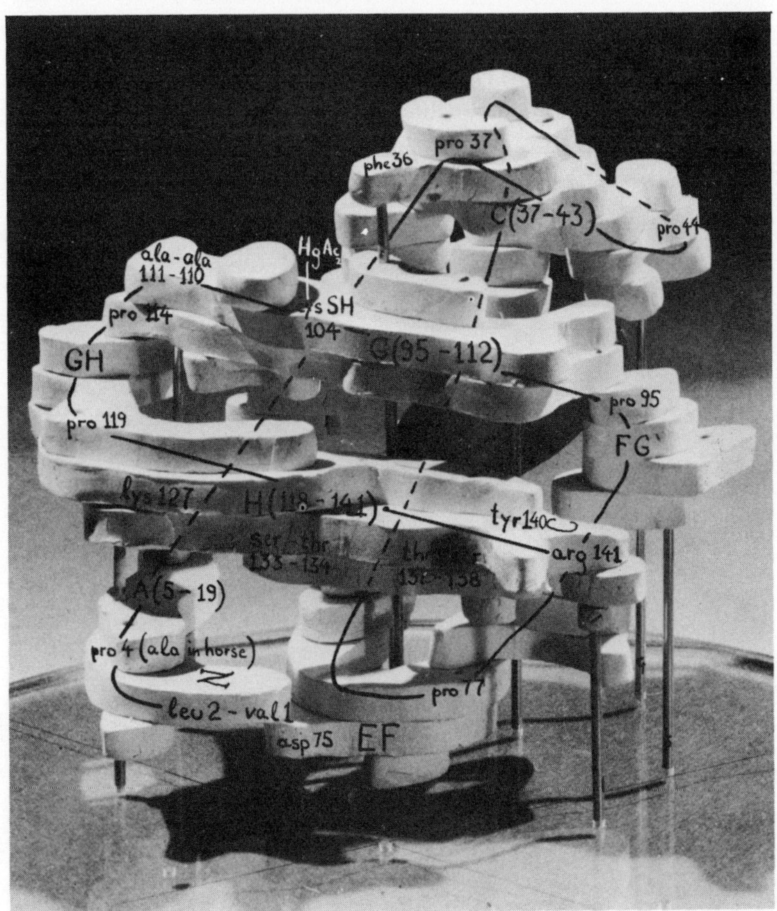

FIGURE 2-3a. Model of the α chain of hemoglobin with some of the amino acid residues from the human α chain
From a photograph kindly supplied by Dr. M. F. Perutz.

chains. This is quite remarkable when it is considered that Kendrew's myoglobin was derived from the sperm whale, whereas Perutz's model was based on horse hemoglobin.

In Figure 2-3, where the complete hemoglobin molecule is shown, we notice also the presence and positioning of the heme groups. These are represented simply as circular discs in the model, showing also the site of attachment of the oxygen molecules. Also visible in this illustration is the beginning of one of the two β peptide chains, the so-called

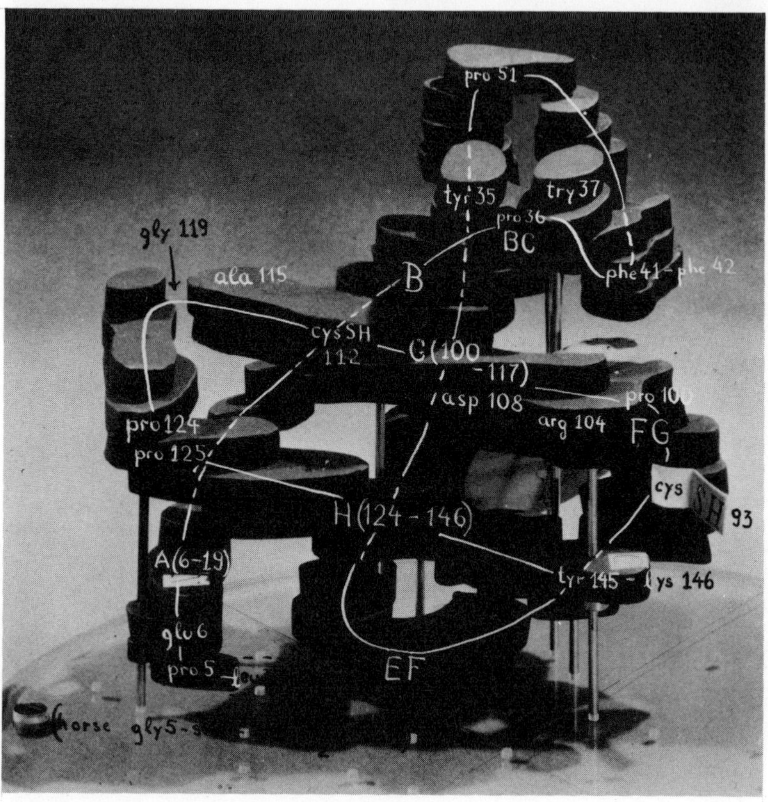

FIGURE 2-3b. Model of the β chain of hemoglobin with some of the amino acid residues of the human β chain
From a photograph kindly supplied by Dr. M. F. Perutz.

N-terminus designated in the figure with N. This is the end of the peptide chain carrying the free amino group of the first amino acid, valine in the case of the α or β chain. The iron atom at the center of each heme group is attached to its particular peptide chain through the side chain of a histidine residue in that chain (see Kendrew *et al.*, 1961). The coordinating position of the iron atom opposite to that linked to histidine is available, when the iron is in the reduced form, for combining with oxygen molecules or with carbon monoxide.

Very recently, Perutz (unpublished) presented data on the structure of deoxygenated human hemoglobin. The evidence from amino acid sequences and from analysis of x-ray structure indicates close similarity between horse and human hemoglobin, so that the deoxygenated form of one may be compared with the oxygenated form of the other. The major change upon deoxygenation appears to be in two of the four polypeptide chains, the so-called beta chains. These two beta chains move out from the center of the molecule and away from each other by a few Angstrom units, thus increasing the distance separating the two heme groups embedded in the beta chains—the point of attachment of the oxygen molecules. There is also a slight change in the angle between two helical portions of the beta peptide chains. These findings represent a great step forward in our understanding of the molecular basis of the most important property of hemoglobin, the ability to combine reversibly with oxygen.

MYOGLOBIN

Figure 2-4 is a representation of the model of myoglobin recently produced by Kendrew (1961). Much detail is visible and in particular most of the amino acid sequence could be determined clearly by x-ray methods. An absolute identification was possible in many cases in spite of the fact that individual atoms were not resolved, since the outline of many amino acid side chains could be distinguished. Only a few ambiguities remained. The amino acid sequences determined in this way agree with those found by orthodox chemical methods (Edmundson and Hirs, 1961). A few features in this very complex model are particularly important. The flat heme group with its iron atom at the center is easily visible; the linkage of the iron atom to the histidine residue F-8 is also clearly visible. There seems to be a space available at the sixth coordination position on the opposite side of this heme group, where normally an oxygen or a carbon monoxide molecule

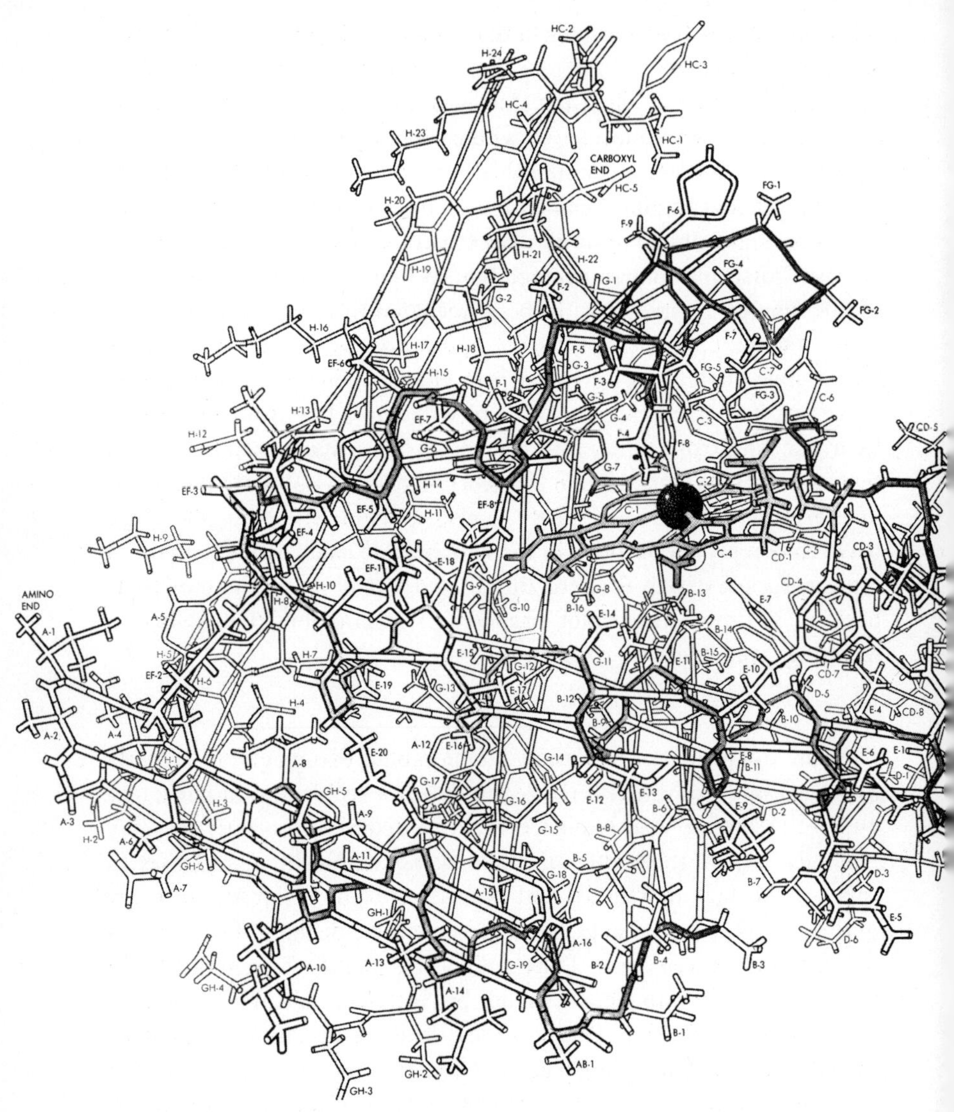

FIGURE 2-4. Model of sperm whale myoglobin
Sperm whale myoglobin showing the three-dimensional arrangement of the single polypeptide chain together with the amino acid sequence. (Kendrew, 1961.)

would coordinate with the iron atom in the usual physiological functioning of myoglobin. There is also a second histidine residue near the sixth position of this iron atom, which is residue E-7, too far away to complex directly with the iron. However, there are certain variants of human *hemoglobin*, the so-called hemoglobins M, in which this particular histidine residue is replaced by the amino acid tyrosine (Gerald and Efron, 1961). The phenolic side chain of this amino acid in its ionized phenolate form is somewhat larger and is able to complex directly with the iron atom. The result is a stable complex with the iron in the ferric form which is stable and physiologically ineffective. We are here, however, taking the liberty of comparing the structure of a human hemoglobin with the structure of the myoglobin peptide chain (Watson and Kendrew, 1961). Nevertheless, everything we know so far about the structures of these two chains leads us to believe that this comparison is really valid.

The beginning of the peptide chain, the end bearing the free amino group, is clearly visible and the continuation of the chain can be traced in Figure 2-4. Those α helices which can be seen have the appearance of long cylinders of peptide chain. Where an α helix ends, and before the next one begins, there is a sequence of amino acids, sometimes short and sometimes long, which has no regular arrangement in space. On the other hand, these link sequences have a configuration which is specific for this part of the myoglobin molecule. The various helices and folds of the peptide chain are not held together by covalent bonds, but by ionic interactions, by van der Waals forces, and by hydrogen bonds. The sequence of amino acids has to be exact if the various interacting groups are to be in their correct positions.

COVALENT STRUCTURE OF THE HEMOGLOBIN PEPTIDE CHAINS

The α peptide chain of human adult hemoglobin has 141 amino acids; the β chain has 146 (Figure 2-5). These two peptide chains (Braunitzer *et al.*, 1961; Konigsberg *et al.*, 1961; Goldstein *et al.*, 1961; Braunitzer and Rudloff, 1962) are arranged side by side in the figure and in such a way as to give the maximum amount of correspondence in sequence between the two chains. Identical amino acids in similar

The α and β Peptide Chains of

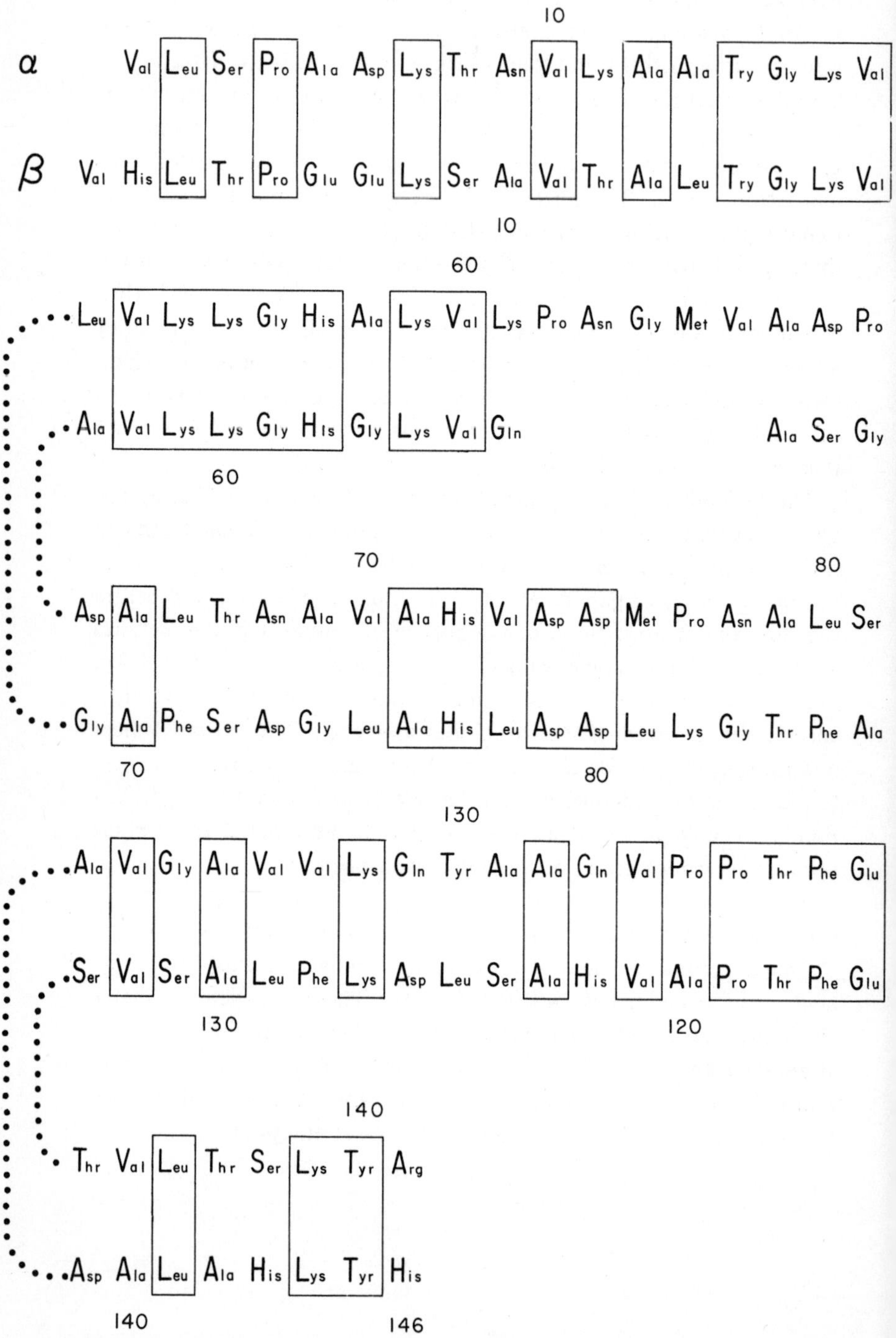

10

α Val Leu Ser Pro Ala Asp Lys Thr Asn Val Lys Ala Ala Try Gly Lys Val

β Val His Leu Thr Pro Glu Glu Lys Ser Ala Val Thr Ala Leu Try Gly Lys Val

10

60

Leu Val Lys Lys Gly His Ala Lys Val Lys Pro Asn Gly Met Val Ala Asp Pro

Ala Val Lys Lys Gly His Gly Lys Val Gln Ala Ser Gly

60

70 80

Asp Ala Leu Thr Asn Ala Val Ala His Val Asp Asp Met Pro Asn Ala Leu Ser

Gly Ala Phe Ser Asp Gly Leu Ala His Leu Asp Asp Leu Lys Gly Thr Phe Ala

70 80

130

Ala Val Gly Ala Val Val Lys Gln Tyr Ala Ala Gln Val Pro Pro Thr Phe Glu

Ser Val Ser Ala Leu Phe Lys Asp Leu Ser Ala His Val Ala Pro Thr Phe Glu

130 120

140

Thr Val Leu Thr Ser Lys Tyr Arg

Asp Ala Leu Ala His Lys Tyr His

140 146

the Human Hemoglobin A

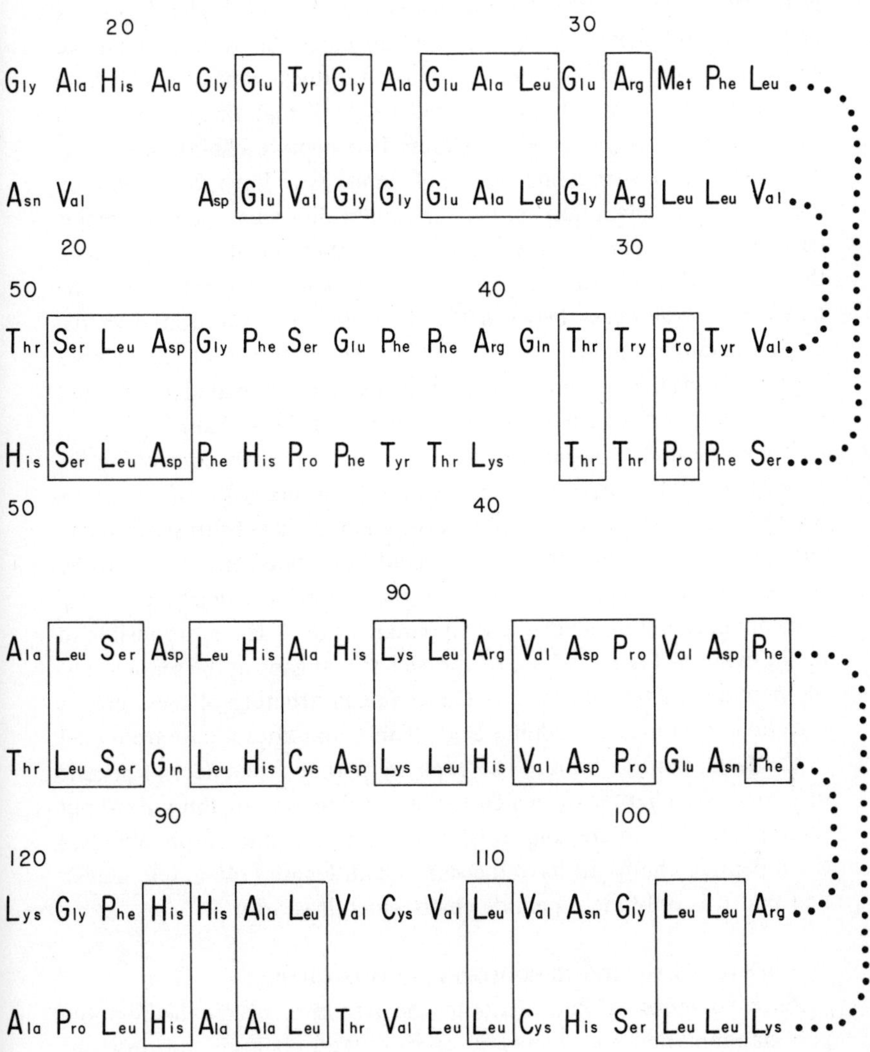

FIGURE 2-5. Sequence of amino acids in the normal human α and β peptide chains

The chains are arranged for maximum homology. Identical residues are enclosed by lines. The apparent "gaps" exist only in the drawing. (Based on the work of Braunitzer, Konigsberg, and colleagues.)

positions in the two chains are indicated in the figure by having a box drawn around them. Altogether we can count 61 pairs of identical amino acids (or about 42 percent of 146 residues), which is a striking degree of similarity. One is tempted to think that there might be a common evolutionary origin for these two peptide chains, since it is hard to visualize such a high degree of similarity to have come about by the convergent evolution of two originally dissimilar peptide chains (see chapter 6). On the other hand, the number of differences between the two chains, namely 85 pairs of amino acids, is greater than the number of differences between the β, γ, and δ chains found in the human hemoglobins A, F (fetal), and A_2. In the family of hemoglobin peptide chains the β, γ, and δ chains are more closely related in structure to one another than any of them are related to the α chain.

The amount of divergence of the two structural genes controlling the α and β chains has presumably come about by a succession of mutations which on the one hand has given rise to amino acid substitutions in one chain or another, and on the other hand has altered the structures by the deletion of genetic material with the consequent deletion of one, two, or more amino acids. The apparent "gaps" which are visible in the drawing of Figure 2-5 are of course not real gaps in the sequence of the peptide chains themselves. The covalent structure of these chains is quite continuous and amino acids before and after a gap are joined in the usual peptide bond. The gaps are perhaps the effect of genetic deletions (see chapter 6), which is the simplest way of thinking about these gaps. It is interesting to note that the β, γ, and (probably also) the δ peptide chains all have the same chain length (146 amino acids), and that it is only the α peptide chain which is shorter.

THE SYNTHESIS OF THE HEMOGLOBIN PEPTIDE CHAINS

Since so much is known about the structure of the hemoglobin peptide chains and since there is a variety of these chains in the molecule, people have readily seen that the hemoglobin system is a useful one for the study of protein synthesis. The hemoglobin system has another advantage which can be utilized in these studies, namely that the immature red cell is a synthetic system, the main product of which is the single protein, hemoglobin. In most microbial systems and in the liver systems for the study of protein synthesis we are always confronted with the difficulty that a mixture of proteins is being made and that this mixture is very hard to separate and characterize chemically. On the other hand, in the hemoglobin system we can study the biosynthesis of specific peptide chains whose structure is largely understood.

In some recent experiments Dintzis (1961) tried to answer the question of whether a peptide chain grows in a linear fashion from one end to the other or whether it might not grow from the middle outwards or in several places at the same time. For his studies Dintzis used rabbit reticulocytes from animals made anemic by the injection of phenylhydrazine. These cells are very active in the synthesis of hemoglobin and they make apparently little else. This fact is rather strange at first sight, because in order to make hemoglobin some other protein enzymes have to be present as well. The mechanism of synthesis requires the presence of amino acid activating enzymes and a whole lot of other enzymes concerned with the synthesis of heme. However, by using a reticulocyte, which is the penultimate stage in the red cell series, most of the enzymes required are already present and very little more is made. In any case these other enzymes only amount to a very few percent of the total protein content of the cell.

Figure 2-6 shows the theoretical model which Dintzis uses as his scheme for the synthesis of soluble hemoglobin. Protein synthesis occurs in the ribosomes which are nucleoprotein particles in the cell. In the case of the reticulocyte, the ribosomes are free and are not attached to an endoplasmic reticulum, as they are in other mammalian cells, such as the liver cells. If we look at a cell and ask: what is the state of the hemoglobin peptide chains in the average ribosome, Dintzis would answer that there will be a distribution of *unfinished* (and unlabeled) peptide chains of varying lengths, as indicated at the top of Figure 2-6 at time t_1. Some chains will have hardly begun to grow, others will be finished, and there will be others of intermediate lengths If at that time one gives a short pulse of radioactive amino acid, for example H^3-leucine, to such a cell, then during that pulse each peptide chain will grow a small length of radioactive peptide chain as shown at time t_2 in Figure 2-6. The length of the pulse at time t_2 is short compared to the time which it takes to make the whole chain. After such a short time interval only a few of the peptide chains will be complete

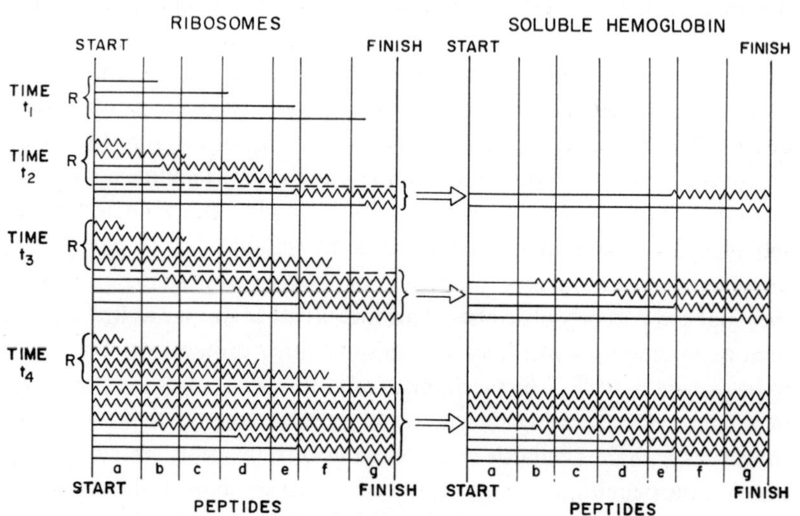

FIGURE 2-6. Model of sequential chain growth

The straight lines represent unlabeled peptide chain. The zigzag lines represent radioactively labeled peptide chain formed after the addition of radioactive amino acid at time t_1. The groups of peptides labeled *R* are those unfinished bits attached to the ribosome at each time; the rest, having reached the finish line, are assumed to be present in the soluble hemoglobin. In the ribosome at time t_2, the top two completely zigzag lines represent peptide chains formed completely from amino acids during the time interval between t_1 and t_2. The middle two lines represent chains which have grown during that time interval, but have not reached the finish line and are therefore still attached to the ribosomes. The bottom two chains represent those which have crossed the finish line, left the ribosomes and are to be found mixed with other molecules of soluble hemoglobin. The symbols a–g indicate the tryptic peptides to be expected. (Dintzis, 1961.)

enough to be released and therefore we will find amongst the soluble hemoglobin molecules some peptide chains which have that portion of the chain labeled which was synthesized last. If we have a means of separating and examining different portions of the peptide chain of the soluble hemoglobin and if we can locate the radioactivity in such portions of the peptide chain, then we can deduce which part of the chain is synthesized last of all. If the length of time of the exposure to radioactive leucine is increased, then each peptide chain will grow more, as shown at time t_3 in Figure 2-6. More and more label will appear in the finished peptide chains of the soluble hemoglobin, until eventually at time t_4 and at longer times label will be distributed more or less evenly throughout the length of the peptide chain.

Dintzis studied the soluble hemoglobin released by the ribosome after pulse experiments with tritiated leucine for various lengths of time. He used trypsin to split the peptide chains into a definite number of small peptides, labeled *a* to *g* in Figure 2-6. These fragments were separated and characterized by paper chromatography and paper electrophoresis—fingerprinting. The figure which is really required in these experiments is the specific activity of leucine in each of the individual peptide fragment $a - g$. However, this is technically difficult to determine when working with small amounts of protein and relatively low levels of radioactivity, because the yield of each peptide fragment is variable from experiment to experiment and also differs from peptide to peptide. An internal standard was desirable, corresponding to the portions of peptide chain made before the pulse began; the radioactivity due to the pulse could then be compared to that standard. Dintzis added carrier hemoglobin at the end of each experiment which was uniformly labeled with radioactive C^{14}-leucine from a long time incubation. The pulse experiment itself was performed with H^3-leucine. At the end of the pulse and after the cells were opened, Dintzis added his uniformly labeled C^{14}-leucine hemoglobin and digested the mixture with trypsin. In each isolated peptide he was then able to determine the ratio of tritium to C^{14} and, since the latter was uniform for each peptide, this ratio gave him a measure of the specific activity of tritium label in each peptide. In fact, before the trypsin digestion, Dintzis isolated the α and β peptide chain on a carboxymethylcellulose-column and then digested the globin from each chain separately.

The kind of data which he obtained is reproduced in Figure 2-7, where it is separately recorded for the α and the β peptide chain. The relative amount of tritium is the measure of label in each peptide acquired during the pulse experiment. The peptide number given in these plots is quite arbitrary, but Dintzis found that he could arrange his data as more or less straight lines by putting these peptides in a sequence of increasing relative tritium radioactivity. At an incubation time of four minutes only the last four peptides received significant amounts of radioactivity, indicating that that end of the chain is made last. On

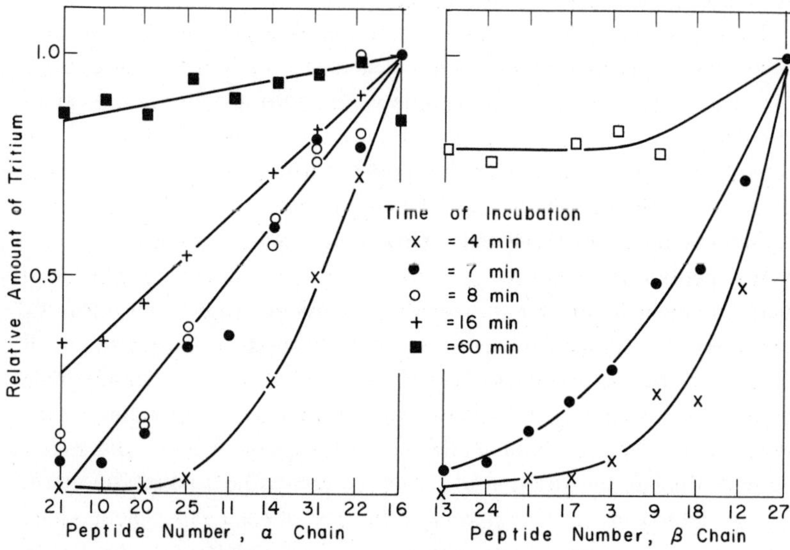

FIGURE 2-7. Distribution of H^3-leucine among tryptic peptides of soluble rabbit hemoglobin after various times of incubation at 15°C
The rate of synthesis is approximately one-fourth of the rate at 37°C. The points at seven minutes are the average of six experiments.

the other hand, seven minutes was evidently enough to complete a whole peptide chain and at 16 minutes more than one chain was made, in other words a new round of synthesis had begun. It should be noted at this point that Dintzis' experiments were done at 15°C in order to slow down sufficiently the rate of synthesis so that early enough samples could be withdrawn. At this temperature he found that the overall rate of the synthesis is about one-fourth of that at 37°C. From this data it appears that one peptide chain is made in about 7 minutes at 15°C or 1.5 minutes at 37°C.

The fact that an approximately linear plot is obtained in the α chain experiments, that for short pulses only the peptides on the right hand side of the figure are labeled, and that at increasing pulse times the slope of the plot becomes almost zero, is in accordance with the model proposed by Dintzis and illustrated in Figure 2-6. The experiments show within the limits of the techniques employed that the chain grows linearly from one end to the other and that the amino acids are added sequentially. However, since only leucine was used in these experiments, we cannot be sure of what happens in the peptide chain sequences between the individual leucine residues. The possibility cannot be ruled out that at certain points in the chain, groups of amino acids are added, although this possibility seems remote.

Dintzis also showed that the hottest amino acid in the α chain (in his peptide number 16) is in fact at the C-terminus. He digested pulse labeled α chains with carboxypeptidases A and B, which liberated arginine and other residues from the C-terminus of that chain and thereby removed Dintzis' peptide 16 from its usual position on the fingerprints. The corresponding experiment with the β chain was not quite so successful. Nevertheless, the experiments indicate that the C-terminal peptide is the last one to be made in the synthesis of at least the α chain and that therefore the growth of the chain begins at the N-terminus and then proceeds along the chain. More recently, Dintzis and Naughton (1962) have compared the amino acid compositions of the tryptic peptides of their rabbit hemoglobin which was used in these experiments with the known compositions of the tryptic peptides of the human α and β chains. There is a very striking degree of similarity between these two sets of peptides which enabled Dintzis and Naughton to assign a provisional *order* for their labeled peptides by assuming a high degree of homology between rabbit hemoglobin and human hemoglobin. The idea that a peptide chain grows linearly from the N-terminus is strengthened, because their purely empirical sequence of peptide numbers in Figure 2-7 is in fact confirmed in every single instance by their new determination of peptide sequence from the analysis of the tryptic peptides. The overall conclusion that the peptide chain grows linearly from the N-terminus was previously reported by Bishop, Leahy, and Schweet (1960) for hemoglobin synthesis; and by Yoshida and Tobita (1960) for bacterial amylase. More recently Anfinsen and his colleagues working with chicken lysozyme (1962) have obtained data similar to that of Dintzis. In particular Anfinsen's data is very convincing, because he was able to combine the results of pulse label experiments with the accurately known positions in the peptide chain of the radioactive amino acid used. We now have a reasonably clear picture of a fundamental aspect of protein synthesis.

Very recently the rather similar experiments of Knopf (1962) in a cell-free system prepared from rabbit reticulocytes have confirmed the results of Dintzis. However, Knopf's system differs not only in being very much less active in hemoglobin synthesis, but also in the inability of his cellfree system to start a new round of synthesis of peptide chains. Knopf finds that his ribosomes are only capable of completing the synthesis of chains already started before their isolation; no new chain formation is begun. This fact and the very much slower rate of synthesis (a fraction of 1 percent) of the cellfree system present a great puzzle. It seems that as soon as the cell is broken and before any of the constituents are fractionated, the rate of synthesis has already fallen to the cell-free level. The explanation for this phenomenon may provide insight into an aspect of protein synthesis about which we know very little—namely, the conditions necessary for the laying down of new peptide chains. In addition we may begin to understand the molecular basis for the need to keep the organization of the cell intact.

THE UNIVERSALITY OF THE PROTEIN SYNTHESIZING MECHANISM

Another experiment, also concerned with the mechanism of hemoglobin biosynthesis, was recently performed by Lipmann and von Ehrenstein (1961) at the Rockefeller Institute. They tested the universality of the protein synthesizing mechanism by reconstituting a cellfree system partly from constituents of rabbit reticulocytes and partly from extracts of *Escherichia coli.* The experiment was a success and they were able to show that rabbit hemoglobin had been synthesized.

One of the intermediates in protein synthesis in bacteria and in mammals is the activated form of the amino acids as an amino acyl-sRNA compound (NH_2·CHR·CO—sRNA). It is in this combination that the amino acids arrive in the ribosome, there to line up on the template and to join into peptide chains. The sRNA (or transfer-RNA, soluble RNA, amino acid acceptor RNA) has a molecular weight of 25,000 – 30,000 with 80 – 100 nucleotides. It is postulated that there is at least one specific type of sRNA molecule for each amino acid and more for some amino acids. The first step in protein synthesis is the activation of the carboxyl group of each amino acid by ATP and a specific activating enzyme to form an aminoacyl-adenylate-enzyme complex. The same enzyme transfers the activated amino acid to the sRNA molecule to form the amino acyl-sRNA compound (see review by Berg, 1961).

Normally in reconstituting a cellfree hemoglobin synthesizing system, the ribosome and also the sRNA and the activating enzymes would all be derived from reticulocytes. Von Ehrenstein and Lipmann labeled *E. coli* sRNA with C^{14}-leucine and the other C^{12}-amino acids, which are required, in the presence of *E. coli* activating enzymes. This preparation when incubated with rabbit ribosomes in a suitable medium was able to transfer over 60 percent of its radioactivity to soluble hemoglobin. The labeled leucine went directly from its compound with sRNA into hemoglobin, without first passing through a pool of free leucine, since the addition of C^{12}-leucine did not affect the yield of labeled hemoglobin. What is more, the authors digested with trypsin the labeled rabbit hemoglobin synthesized in this experiment. A fingerprint of the tryptides obtained showed a high degree of correspondence between the ninhydrin positive peptides (old hemoglobin made in the rabbit) and those visible in the radioautogram (freshly synthesized hemoglobin). This almost exact matching of spots gives one great confidence that the cellfree reticulocyte system really made hemoglobin with its leucine residues in their correct positions. Therefore, at least the leucine-specific sRNA from *E. coli* carries the same recognition sites for the ribosomal template as does the reticulocyte sRNA. Possibly, the same holds true for the rest of the *E. coli* sRNA molecules, although recent experiments by Benzer and Weisblum

(1961) suggest species differences might exist between some of the sRNA's of rabbit, yeast, and *E. coli* with respect to their interaction with the activating enzymes.

More recently, von Ehrenstein (unpublished) showed that *E. coli* cysteine-specific sRNA carried its C^{14}-labeled amino acid into the correct place on the rabbit hemoglobin template so that the amino acid, cysteine, appeared in the appropriate peptides. The sulfur in this cysteinyl-sRNA compound was removed chemically with Raney nickel, so that the amino acid was now actually alanine, but still attached to cysteine-specific sRNA. The rabbit hemoglobin made with this material, together with the other C^{12}-aminoacyl-sRNA compounds, had C^{14}-alanine in peptides which normally contain cysteine but not alanine. This is a striking demonstration of the fact that once an amino acid is attached to its appropriate sRNA the placement of this amino acid on the template is solely a function of the sRNA.

3

THE QUALITATIVE CONTROL OF PROTEIN STRUCTURE: ABNORMAL HEMOGLOBINS

Since it would take far too long to give a comprehensive account of the chemical work on the abnormal human hemoglobins, we will confine ourselves to discussing a selection of abnormalities. These are chemical changes in the hemoglobin molecule which are genetically determined and which are thought to be due to mutations in the hemoglobin gene. In the most recent review on the subject, Baglioni (1962) lists 34 electrophoretic variants of hemoglobin A in which the peptide chain (α or β) carrying the abnormality is known. In 15 of these hemoglobins the particular amino acid substitution has been identified and located exactly at a certain residue position in the peptide chain. Most of the chemical work was done in the last six years, although some of it goes back to the original electrophoretic characterization of sickle-cell anemia hemoglobin (S) by Pauling and Itano in 1949. It might be instructive to review briefly the history of this first abnormal hemoglobin.

SICKLE-CELL ANEMIA AND ITS HEMOGLOBIN

Even today sickle-cell anemia is the best studied example of an inherited disease in which one can point clearly to the molecular basis for the disease and its symptoms. The occurrence of sickled erythrocytes in this anemia was first described by Herrick in 1910. Two kinds of individuals were found in whom sickling of erythrocytes could be induced by reducing the oxygen tension of a sample of blood: those which were apparently healthy (carriers of sickle cell trait) and a few others who had a severe hemolytic anemia. The sickling phenomenon was recognized as an inherited condition by Taliafero and Huck in 1923, who considered it to be a dominant Mendelian character, taking both sickle cell anemia and the largely asymptomatic sickle cell trait as variable expressions of the same abnormal gene. In 1949, Neel and Beet, independently, put forward the now accepted view that individuals with the severe sickle cell anemia were homozygous for an abnormal gene and that sickle-cell trait carriers were heterozygous, having one normal and one abnormal gene. Whether this genetic character is to be described as codominant, dominant, or recessive depends on how one defines it. If one looks for the production of an abnormal hemoglobin protein, than the two genes producing Hb A and Hb S are codominant, since each produces its characteristic gene product; the heterozygote has both hemoglobins (A and S) in its blood. If the descriptive characteristic of the phenotype is the presence of a positive sickling test on that person's blood, then the "Hb S gene" is dominant, since both the heterozygote and the homozygote give this test. Thirdly, if the clinical picture of sickle-cell anemia is taken as the distinguishing criterion, then the "Hb S gene" is recessive, since only the homozygote has the disease and since the heterozygote has only the trait.

The reason for the sickling of deoxygenated red cells containing sickle-cell hemoglobin (S) was obscure until Harris (1950) showed the presence of birefringent bodies in deoxygenated solutions of this hemoglobin. Next, Perutz, and Mitchison (1951) demonstrated the very low solubility of reduced hemoglobin S in salt solutions. We can now see the reason for the sickling phenomenon: the hemoglobin S in the red cell remains in solution as the normally soluble oxyhemoglobin S as long as the cells are in an oxygen rich environment. When the partial pressure of oxygen is reduced, either artificially or in the tissues, the hemoglobin protein inside the cell precipitates to form paracrystalline aggregates or tactoids which distort the cell to the sickle-cell shape. This is apparently not true crystallization, but rather the aggregates are bundles of two-dimensional arrays of molecules (see Allison,

Scientific American, 1956). Although we know now the chemical alteration which characterizes hemoglobin S, the chemical and structural explanation of the low solubility of this molecule still escapes us. It remains to be seen, whether all aspects of the clinical picture of sickle-cell anemia can be explained solely in terms of the chemical abnormality of the hemoglobin S molecule or whether there is also some interaction of the chemically abnormal protein with other factors. For the purposes of our discussion, however, we will take the view that the disease is due to the chemical abnormality of the hemoglobin.

The red cells in sickle-cell trait can also be made to sickle in the laboratory, if oxygen is deliberately removed from the sample, or *in vivo* at high altitudes or during flights in unpressurized aircraft. In the people who have the trait (heterozygotes Hb A/Hb S) and who have both hemoglobins, nearly all the cells can be made to sickle (Itano *et al.*, 1956; Itano, 1960). Presumably then, each cell contains both hemoglobin A and S. The alternative situation, that there are cells with hemoglobin A and other cells with hemoglobin S can be ruled out, since in that case only half the cells could be made to sickle. This is an important point; both members of the allelic pair are active within the same cell.

The fact that only hemoglobin A ($\alpha_2^A\beta_2^A$) and hemoglobin S ($\alpha_2^A\beta_2^S$) are found in the heterozygous cell is curious and needs an explanation. One might have expected the formation of a "hybrid" molecule, $\alpha_2^A\beta^A\beta^S$, which would easily be detected. However, this is not the case (Itano, 1960); we must infer that β^A and β^S peptide chains are made in separate places in the cell, perhaps in different ribosomes, and that they dimerize ($2\beta^A \rightarrow \beta_2^A$; $2\beta^S \rightarrow \beta_2^S$) before they are liberated into a common pool. From this it is only one further step to the view that individual ribosomes contain only a single template or at least the templates from only one structural gene, because a compartmentalization of the ribosome is difficult to accept.

The proportion of hemoglobin S in A/S heterozygotes varies from about 25 percent to over 40 percent (see Figure 3-6; Wells and Itano, 1951). The fact that the phenotype of the heterozygote expresses the genotype relatively faithfully has made the abnormal hemoglobin a particularly attractive field for those who wish to study the chemical effects of gene mutations on the structure of a protein molecule.

It was clear by 1954 that the chemical difference between hemoglobin A and S was a small one. Careful quantitative amino acid analyses of the two proteins had shown differences so small as to be indistinguishable from the experimental error of the methods used. In a molecule like hemoglobin, in which each of the identical halves contains some 280 amino acid residues of 19 different kinds, we can expect that many amino acids will occur in more than 15 moles per half molecule. Even the best method of analysis has an error 2–3 percent, which is approaching half of a residue or more of the common amino acids. Single amino acid substitutions amongst those would not be easily detected. Of course, other amino acids are rare; a change of one such might be noticeable.

It was likely from Pauling and Itano's work that an amino acid with a charged side chain was involved in the alteration and that glutamic acid, aspartic acid, lysine, histidine, or arginine might be involved. These all occur sufficiently frequently, except for arginine, to make analysis of the total hydrolysate an unreliable tool for the detection of the appearance or disappearance of one of these amino acids. It turned out (Ingram, 1957) that a glutamic acid has disappeared from hemoglobin A, to be replaced by the even more common amino acid valine in hemoglobin S or by the common amino acid lysine in hemoglobin C (Hunt and Ingram, 1958). An increase in lysine in hemoglobin C had been reported by Huismann *et al.* (1955), but together with other amino acid changes which so far have not been confirmed.

Numerous attempts were made to try and pinpoint the chemical difference between the hemoglobins A and S. Murayama (1958) found that the available sulfhydryl groups (and other silver binding groups) of reduced hemoglobin A varied in number with the temperature. For example, at 0°C he could measure by titration with $Ag(NH_3)_2^+$ that there were four groups capable of binding silver and at 38°C that there were three groups. However, with hemoglobin S there were four and two silver binding groups at these two temperatures, respectively. This is a sensitive method for probing the architecture of the protein molecule, since differences measured by Murayama are likely to be differences in accessibility of the —SH group to the attacking reagent—the silver ammine ion. In turn, accessibility depends upon the configuration of the polypeptide chains rather than on the primary amino acid sequences of the chain. It is not likely that the actual number of sulfhydryl groups in the peptide chains of the two hemoglobins differs in view of the titration results of other people and the careful amino acid analyses for cysteine by Stein *et al.* (1957). We do not know the chemical nature of the other silver binding groups.

The two hemoglobins were indistinguishable by the x-ray crystallographic techniques available to Perutz *et al.* in 1951. They formed the same series of crystal forms with the exception of one new oxyhemoglobin form of hemoglobin S. Of course the reduced hemoglobin S formed crystals which were different from crystals of reduced hemoglobin A, as was to be expected from the altered solubility of reduced hemoglobin S. Crystals of several forms of oxyhemoglobins A and S gave identical x-ray diffraction patterns, a finding which implies that the gross structure of the two molecules is similar. Perutz's result was an important one, because following the demonstration of an electrophoretic difference between hemoglobins A and S the possibility existed that this was due, not to a change in amino acid sequence, but solely to a rearrangement of the same peptide chain in a different folding so as to uncover or to mask charged groups in the protein molecule. The x-ray result makes this possibility unlikely or at any rate restricts a change in folding to such small dimensions, that it would not be able to cover up or uncover charged groups. The fact that an amino acid substitution involving a charged group was actually found does not, of course, preclude the additional possibility, or the likelihood, of a small "disturbance" of the folding of the peptide chains. Only when the three-dimensional structure of these hemoglobins is understood, will the full structural implications of the amino acid substitution be clear.

It was shown by Havinga and Itano (1953) that the heme groups of hemoglobin S were in each case formed as usual by iron in coordination with protoporphyrin IX and that therefore the difference must reside in the protein. The spectra of the two hemoglobins are closely similar. Their oxygen dissociation curves are said to resemble one another, but this seems unlikely on purely physical ground and should be reinvestigated. It does not seem reasonable that a property like oxygen affinity could be unaffected by a change in the molecule which alters the solubility so profoundly and in a way which depends on its state of oxygenation. Some recent experiments by Riggs and Wells (1961) seem to point to a somewhat lower oxygen affinity for hemoglobin S.

The N-terminal amino acids of hemoglobins A and S were found to be valine in both cases by Havinga (1953) and by Huisman and Drinkwaard (1955). The latter also showed that attack on the C-terminal amino acid of the peptide chains of the two proteins with the enzyme carboxypeptidase A liberated from both only histidine and tyrosine. Carboxypeptidase A splits off amino acids one by one beginning from the C-terminal end of a peptide chain, but the speed at which it does so depends on the nature of the particular amino acid and on the one immediately preceding it. We now know that histidine and tyrosine are the last and the penultimate amino acid, respectively, of the β chain. The α chain ends in -tyrosyl-arginine and arginine is not attacked by carboxypeptidase A. For our present purpose it is enough to say that hemoglobin A and S behaved identically.

We may summarize these investigations by concluding that there seemed to be a definite chemical difference between hemoglobins A and S expressed as a change in electrophoretic mobility and that this was likely to be a small one.

FINGERPRINTING

Beyond the identification by electrophoresis of hemoglobins A and S and any other of the abnormal hemoglobins (Figures 3-1, 3-2) further chemical investigation may be carried out in a variety of ways. The proteins can be subjected to a detailed analysis of their spectra, to a determination of their shape in the ultracentrifuge, to studies of their antigenic properties and to a titration of their acidic and basic groups, to mention only a few. However, since it seems likely that inherited abnormalities of the protein reside in an alteration of the primary covalent structure of that protein, it is most important to concentrate on at least a partial elucidation of that primary structure. Again there are many approaches possible, but the one which is most in favor among

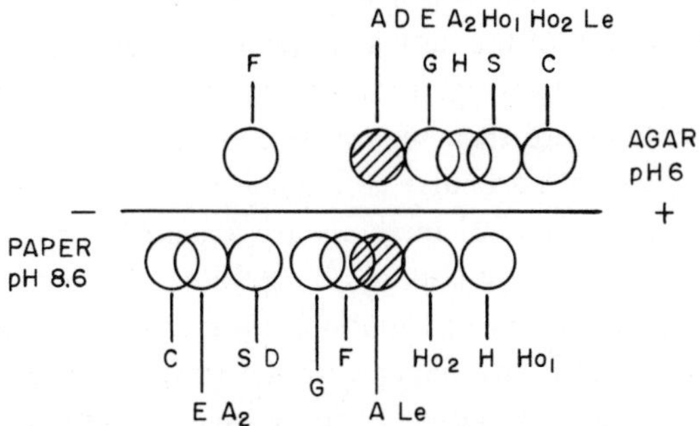

FIGURE 3-1. Migration of human hemoglobins in agar gel (pH ca. 6) and paper (pH 8.6) electrophoresis
Ho_1 = Hb Hopkins-1; Ho_2 = Hb Hopkins-2; Le = Hb Lepore.

protein chemists is a splitting of the peptide chains by specific enzymes which hydrolyze at specific positions in the peptide chains. In the case of the hemoglobins it may or may not be necessary to separate first the individual α and β peptide chains as was done by Dintzis in the

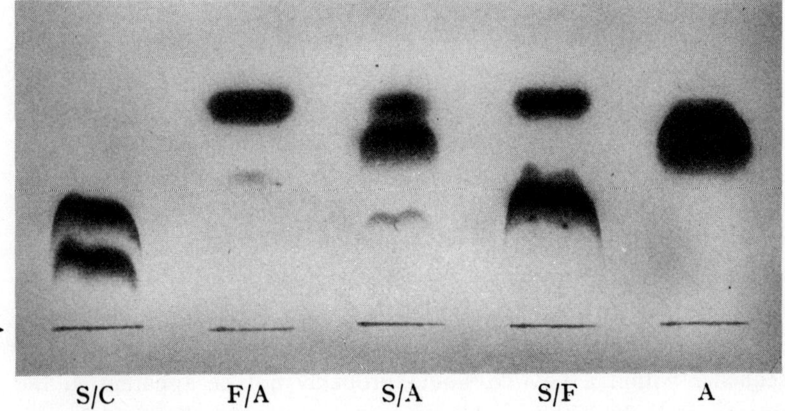

FIGURE 3-2. Drawing of agar gel electrophoresis patterns of mixtures of human hemoglobins (pH 6.2; 0.05 M citrate)

experiments mentioned in the previous chapter. Such a preliminary step results of course in a simpler mixture of peptide fragments to be investigated, but the necessity for chain separation depends upon the resolution of the method which is going to be used for the isolation and characterization of the individual peptide fragments.

Following the initial digestion of the protein or peptide chain, individual peptides are then separated and investigated more closely as to their content of particular amino acids and as to the sequence of these amino acids. Several methods are available for the separation and characterization of mixtures of peptides. Among these can be mentioned countercurrent distribution, ion exchange chromatography, paper electrophoresis, and paper chromatography. The combination of these last two methods has been the choice in the author's laboratory. The technique has come to be known as fingerprinting; it is a combination of the methods originally developed by Sanger (summarized by Harris and Ingram, 1960) and also by Knight (1954). Figure 3-3a shows two fingerprints of hemoglobin A and hemoglobin S (Ingram, 1958; Baglioni, 1961). In each case the peptide mixture obtained by trypsin digestion of whole hemoglobin is separated first by paper electrophoresis at pH 6.4, followed by ascending paper chromatography at right angles to the direction of electrophoresis on the same sheet of paper. For close comparison two digests are run side by side in both these operations. As the Figure shows, the various peptide fragments are located in definite and characteristic positions in these fingerprints, so that the whole digest results in a characteristic pattern or fingerprint. To a considerable extent this pattern reflects the amino acid sequences to be found in the individual peptides and therefore the covalent primary structure of the hemoglobin molecules. Like all other techniques, fingerprinting has its limitations, being especially sensitive to changes in charged amino acids and less sensitive to alterations involving uncharged groups. In particular an inversion of amino acid sequence within a peptide would probably not be apparent in the fingerprint, unless the inversion happened to span a cleavage site, such as a lysine or arginine residue, or unless it happened to alter the sensitivity to trypsin of a lysine or arginine residue next to it. In addition it

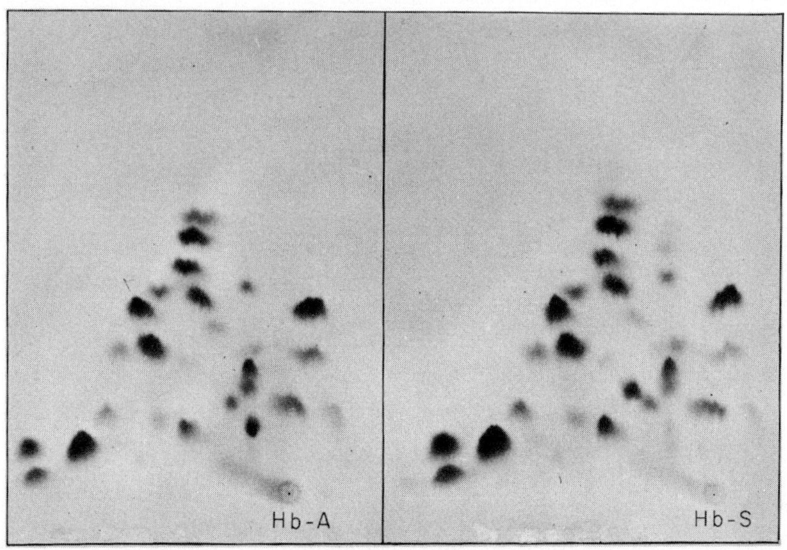

FIGURE 3-3a. Fingerprints of hemoglobins A and S
Photograph of ninhydrin positive spots. (Baglioni, 1961.)

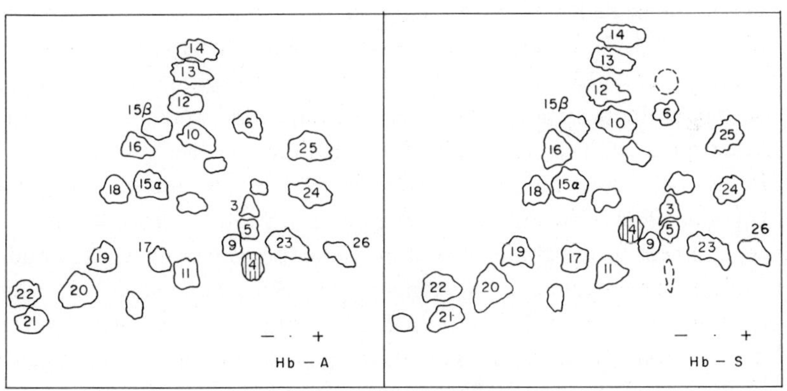

FIGURE 3-3b. Fingerprints of hemoglobins A and S
Tracing of Figure 3-3a showing old numbering system. (Baglioni, 1961.)

is necessary to establish that individual spots on the fingerprint represent single peptides and it will be found that some spots contain several peptides. In such a case it will always be necessary to elute from the fingerprint and investigate the constituents of such multiple spots under different conditions before a definitive comparison between the parent proteins can be made.

In Figure 3-3a it can be easily seen that the two fingerprints are largely identical and further it could be shown that such spots as were multiple contained in both cases the correct number of peptides. Furthermore, identical spots, contained semiquantitatively the same amino acids. There is however one single peptide which assumes a new and different position in sickle cell hemoglobin. It is electrophoretically different from the corresponding hemoglobin A peptide and it also differs in its position in the chromatography direction. The hemoglobin S peptide has clearly lost at least one (net) negative charge which represents a chemical alteration in line with that observed by Pauling and Itano for the whole hemoglobin molecule. Due to the symmetry of the molecule any chemical change is found twice in a whole molecule; it follows that the minimum alteration in the hemoglobin molecule must be two charge units as indeed was calculated by Itano (1957). In Figure 3-4 are shown the amino acid sequences of the peptide spot which was found to differ in the fingerprints of hemoglobin A and S. It turns out that this is an octapeptide which is in fact the first peptide of the β chain of hemoglobin at the N-terminus—number 4 in the old nomenclature and peptide βT I in the new (Gerald and Ingram, 1961). The difference between these peptides turns out to be a replacement of the glutamic acid in the sixth position of the β peptide chain of hemoglobin A by valine in the sickle cell hemoglobin. This exchange explains the loss of the negative charge as well as the difference in the chromatographic mobility of the peptide since an extra ionizable glutamic acid group in the hemoglobin A peptide will tend to slow down the mobility in the basic chromatographic solvent system which is used. So far this particular amino acid change has been found by at least two other investigators (Hill and Schwartz, 1959; Jones and Schroeder, unpublished) and in five different samples of sickle cell hemoglobin from different parts of the world (Ingram, 1959b). Investigation of the remaining peptides by total amino acid analysis and of that portion of the hemoglobin molecule which does not appear in these fingerprints (about one-third of the protein, the so-called "core," Hunt and Ingram, 1958) has shown no changes in the primary structure elsewhere in the molecule within the limits set by the techniques. A really

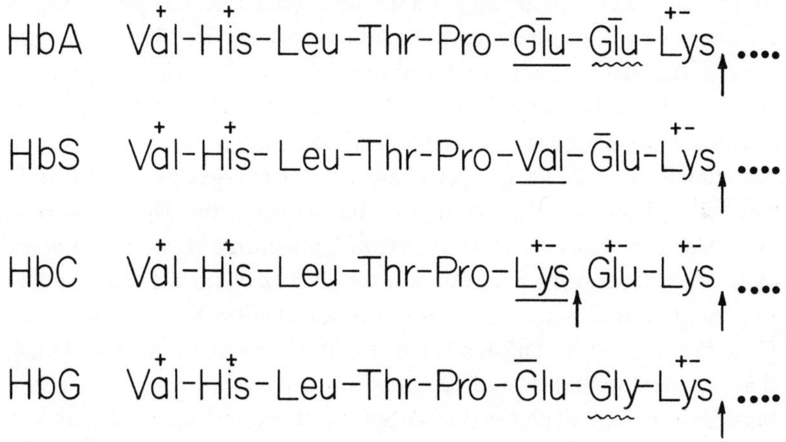

HbA Val-His-Leu-Thr-Pro-Glu-Glu-Lys ....

HbS Val-His-Leu-Thr-Pro-Val-Glu-Lys ....

HbC Val-His-Leu-Thr-Pro-Lys Glu-Lys ....

HbG Val-His-Leu-Thr-Pro-Glu-Gly-Lys ....

FIGURE 3-4. Sequence of the peptides 4 (βTpI) of hemoglobins A, S, C, and $G_{\text{San José}}$

definite answer to the question of whether the glutamic acid to valine exchange is indeed the only alteration in the protein molecule must await the determination of the complete amino acid sequence of the β peptide chains of sickle-cell hemoglobin. Nevertheless, we will assume for the time being that the only effect of the gene mutation is this single amino acid substitution. We may therefore write a formula for hemoglobin S: $\alpha_2^A\beta_2^{6\ Val}$ (Gerald and Ingram, 1961). This formula indicates that the α chains of sickle-cell hemoglobin are normal, but that position number 6 of the β chain carries valine instead of its usual glutamic acid. It is not at all clear why such an amino acid substitution should produce the drastic change in solubility of the whole molecule (Perutz and Mitchison, 1950) to which has been ascribed the origin of the sickle-cell anemia itself.

HEMOGLOBIN C

It turned out that in hemoglobin C (Itano and Neel, 1950) the same tryptic peptide also showed an alteration in the fingerprint pattern (Hunt and Ingram, 1959b). In fact, it was replaced in the hemoglobin C fingerprints by two new peptides which together had the structure shown in the third line in Figure 3-4. Two new peptides are found, because in the case of hemoglobin C a new lysine residue appears which creates a new bond sensitive to the action of trypsin. Therefore, two peptide fragments result instead of one from the first eight residues of the β chain of hemoglobin C (see Figure 3-4). In hemoglobin C at position 6 of the β chain glutamic acid has been replaced by lysine, a net change of +2 charges per chain or +4 charges per hemoglobin molecule. Therefore the electrophoretic change of the whole protein is expected to be twice as great as that of hemoglobin S, as indeed is the case. The fact that the same 6th position of the β chain has also mutated in hemoglobin C is very good evidence for allelism between the S and C mutations. This confirms the previous proposal by Ranney (1954) that the hemoglobin S and C mutations are allelic, based on several families in whom all children of an S/C heterozygote and a normal A/A parent had one or other, but never both (and never neither) abnormality. Whether the two allelic mutations have arisen independently or whether hemoglobin C is a mutation of the more frequently occurring hemoglobin S gene is, of course, not known.

HEMOGLOBIN $G_{\text{San José}}$

Also shown in Figure 3-4 in the last line is the amino acid sequence of the first eight residues of hemoglobin G, or to be more precise, hemoglobin $G_{\text{San José}}$. This is one of the rare hemoglobins known so far only in one particular family first described by Schwartz *et al.* (1957). From the fingerprints and from sequence determination of the altered peptide (Hill and Schwartz, 1959), it was found that the glutamic acid residue in position 7 of the β chain had been replaced in this particular hemoglobin G by glycine which again results in the loss of a single negative charge in the β chain. Hemoglobin $G_{\text{San José}}$ may therefore be formulated as $\alpha_2^A\beta_2^{7\,\text{Gly}}$. This mutation is not quite a true allele of the hemoglobin S or C mutation, but rather a pseudoallele. Due to the limitations of human genetics it would behave as an allele in family studies, although there is not evidence in this particular family for or against allelism of G and S (Hill *et al.*, 1960) in spite of the fact that both abnormalities occur in the same family. It is interesting to note that the gene mutations which we are discussing here affect only single amino acids and can distinguish quite clearly between neighboring amino acids in a long sequence of 146 residues. The chemical effect of this type of gene mutation is seen to be very specific, precise, and restricted in its action. Why the introduction of a neutral residue in position 7 does not lead to the reduced solubility of the hemoglobin and to the sickling phenomenon as does the introduction of the neutral residue in position 6 of Hb S is still a mystery. This shows in turn how important this particular amino acid sequence is to the functioning of the whole hemoglobin molecule. Finally it is worth noting that in the family already mentioned (Schwartz *et al.*, 1957; Hill *et al.*, 1960) there are two individuals who have only hemoglobin $G_{\text{San José}}$ in their blood due to the simultaneous presence of a (β chain) thalassemia gene which suppresses apparently the formation of hemoglobin A. In spite of the fact that only the abnormal human hemoglobin G is present, these two women do not show clinical symptoms of abnormality as they would do if they had only hemoglobin S. They also have no fetal hemoglobin as is the case with people who possess only hemoglobin S. It seems therefore that hemoglobin $G_{\text{San José}}$ is not deleterious.

DISTRIBUTION OF THE ABNORMALITIES AND BALANCED POLYMORPHISM

The largest number of people with sickle-cell anemia are found in Central and West Africa, although a few other areas also show considerable numbers of this gene. Among the latter, illustrated in Figure 3-5, is the central Mediterranean area, the Persian Gulf, and India. The highest frequencies of the hemoglobin S gene are in areas where tertian malaria was or is endemic. Some time ago Allison (1954), elaborating an earlier idea of Haldane (1949), postulated that the heterozygote for the sickle cell gene was more resistant to this form of malaria than a normal person and in particular that such a heterozygote had fewer malarial parasites in his blood. A direct attempt by Beutler *et al.* (1955) to duplicate Allison's experimental malaria infection in A/A and A/S individuals gave results which did not support the hypothesis. After some controversy about the evidence presented, Allison's view

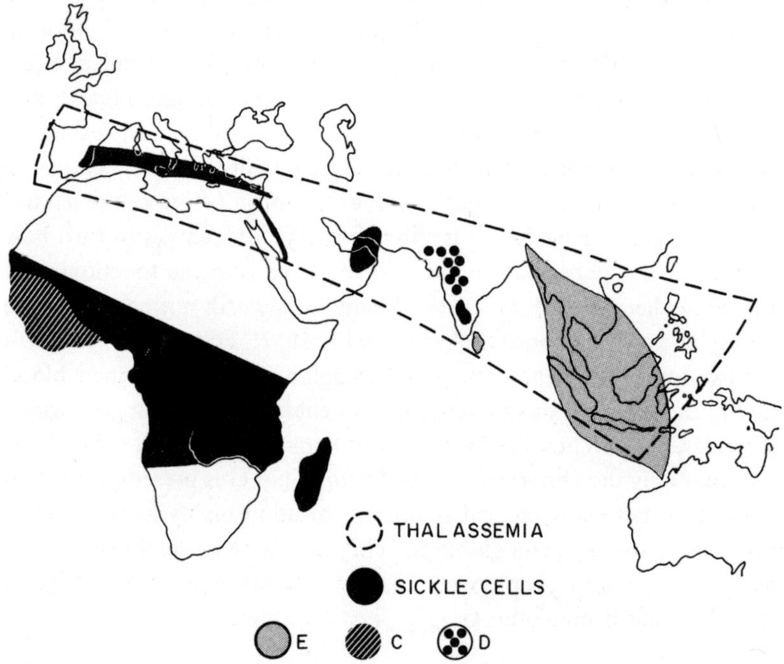

FIGURE 3-5. World distribution of the major hemoglobin abnormalities

By permission from H. Lehmann and J. A. M. Ager, "The hemoglobinopathies and thalassemia," in J. B. Stanbury, J. B. Wyngaarden, and D. S. Fredrickson, eds., *The Metabolic Basis of Inherited Disease* (New York, McGraw-Hill Book Company, Inc., 1960).

has now been accepted (discussed in Rucknagel and Neel, 1961, p. 205). It is especially in the early years of life (Allison, 1957) that malaria is a very killing condition in these parts of Africa and it is at this time that heterozygosity for the sickle-cell gene protects. Raper (1956) has published evidence in support of the idea of balanced polymorphism

TABLE 3-1

INCIDENCE OF SICKLE-CELL TRAIT AMONG ADMISSIONS TO A CHILDREN'S WARD*

Disease group	*Total number*	*Sickle-cell trait*	*Incidence of sickle-cell trait*
Miscellaneous	186	25	0.13
Pneumonia	118	18	0.15
Upper respiratory infections	59	13	0.22
Diarrhea and vomiting	106	25	0.24
Poliomyelitis	26	4	0.15
Tuberculosis	37	8	0.22
Meningitis (purulent)	26	5	0.19
Malnutrition	77	11	0.14
Hookworm anemia	30	2	0.07
Typhoid fever	17	6	0.35
Malaria (a) uncomplicated	83	13	0.16
(b) cerebral	47	—	0
(c) blackwater fever	6	—	0
Total admissions	6	130	0.16
Sickle-cell anemia	31	—	—

* Source: Raper, 1956.

with malaria as the balancing condition. As shown in Table 3-1, taken from Raper, the incidence of sickle cell trait among 818 children admitted to hospital during a certain time period was largely uniform for various admitting diseases, but was zero in a group of forty-seven children suffering from cerebral malaria. These results indicate that sicklers (A/S heterozygous children) were less susceptible to cerebral malaria and therefore possessed a selective advantage.

We seem to have here an explanation of why this gene for sickle cell anemia is so frequent in these areas, in spite of the fact that a considerable number of sickle-cell genes are lost in every generation due to the lethal nature of the homozygous condition in Africa. This state of so-called balanced polymorphism is a good example of this genetic phenomenon.

Hemoglobin C also reaches quite high frequencies in West Africa (see in Lehmann and Ager, 1960), but it is much more restricted in its distribution, seeming to arise from a focus in Ghana. Hemoglobin E is very frequent in South East Asia, including the Veddas of Ceylon. Hemoglobin D is found in India where over a million people seem to possess this gene. The two particular forms of D in India are hemoglobin D_{Punjab} and hemoglobin D_{β} (see later). Whether or not malaria is also involved in causing the high frequencies of these hemoglobin abnormalities is not known. Of course for hemoglobin C, D, and E the disadvantageous nature of the gene is not nearly so high as it is for sickle cell anemia. Even in the homozygous condition these genes are not nearly as deleterious. Therefore, we assume that the selective advantage needed to increase these gene frequencies need not be so high either.

Recently the suggestion has been made by Roberts and Boyo (1960) and also by Firschein (1961) that marriages between a hemoglobin A homozygote and a heterozygote of the AS or the AC type are more fertile and in particular that the number of pregnancies in such matings is somewhat higher for the heterozygote mating. As a consequence the number of live births is higher in such instances, although not as much higher as the number of pregnancies, giving an overall selective advantage to the heterozygote. In addition, it seems from Roberts and Boyo's paper that a child heterozygous for A/S, and even more a child who is A/C, has a better chance of surviving the first few years of life. Although the data of Roberts and Boyo, working with the Yoruba in Southern Nigeria, are indicative of a general trend in the directions just indicated, they are not statistically significant. Firschein's findings, however, are more definite. Among the Black Caribs of British Honduras, with twenty-three percent sickle-cell trait, the fertility ratio of A/S mothers to A/A normals is about 1.45, an impressively high number. It is hard to see at the moment just what the basis for these facts might be and why, for example, a heterozygous mother should show a great number of pregnancies, but the data, particularly in Firschein's paper, are rather convincing.

We have then two groups of explanations for the unexpectedly high frequency of the sickle cell gene (see also as general reference: Rucknagel and Neel, 1961):

Differential mortality. Increased resistance of A/S heterozygotes to *P. falciparum* malaria in first few years of life; fewer parasites in A/S heterozygotes; effect perhaps counterbalanced to a slight degree by a somewhat higher death rate of A/S heterozygous adults (discussed in Rucknagel and Neel, 1961, p. 209); higher birthweight of children born to A/S mothers vs. parasitized A/A mothers; differential mortality perhaps due to shortened life span of A/S erythrocyte or to preferential sickling of parasitized red cells with consequent destruction of such cells and their parasites; no evidence that this effect is operative for Hb C, E or D_{Punjab}.

Differential fertility. Greater number of pregnancies from A/A × A/S matings, particularly if the mother is the heterozygote; consequently elevated number of live births to heterozygous mother, in spite of somewhat increased intrauterine death rate; decreased danger of abortion in A/S mother compared with A/A mother suffering from *P. falciparum;* greater life expectancy in first few years of life for A/S and especially for A/C heterozygous offspring, (same as increased resistance to malaria?); effect is even more marked for A/C heterozygotes, thus providing basis for the high gene frequencies for hemoglobin C.

Wells and Itano (1951) noted some curious aspects of the expression of the sickle-cell gene in heterozygotes of the type A/S in whom they measured accurately the proportion of hemoglobin S to hemoglobin A. If each of the two genes made exactly the same amount of protein, then there would be a fifty : fifty ratio of the two hemoglobins; but this was not the case. In a graphical representation of their data, where the number of individuals is plotted against the percentage of the abnormal hemoglobin (S), as in Figure 3-6, we see that there is a bimodal distribution of frequencies. The means of these two distributions seem to lie at about 42 percent of hemoglobin S and at approximately 35 percent of hemoglobin S. The proportions remained the same for a given individual for samples taken at different times; there was no correlation with sex, age, or different geographical location in the United States. Furthermore, it appeared (Neel *et al.*, 1951) that

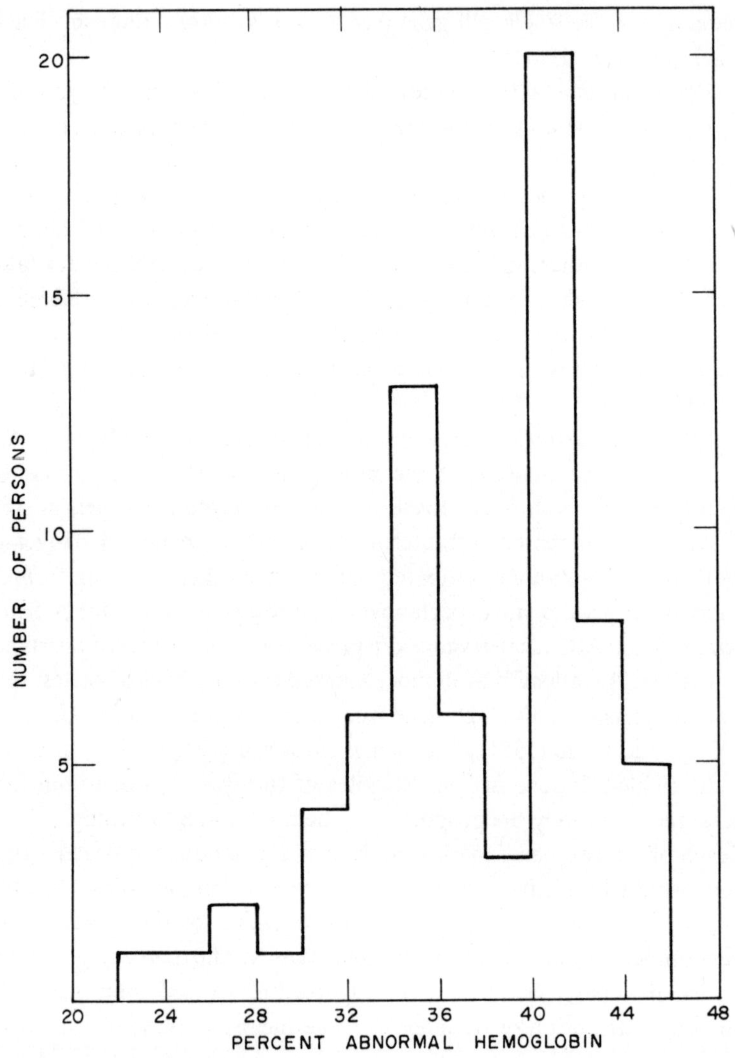

FIGURE 3-6. Distribution of the proportion of hemoglobin S in A/S heterozygotes
(Neel *et al.*, 1951.)

the possession of a high or a low proportion of hemoglobin S was to some extent familial. On the other hand, these authors showed that heterozygotes for hemoglobin S and C showed no such bimodal distribution, but rather that they made equal amounts of the two hemoglobins. Wells and Itano postulated that while the hemoglobin S and C genes cause the manufacture of the same amounts of hemoglobin, there exist at least two different alleles, "isoalleles," of hemoglobin A making proteins indistinguishable by their techniques, but in different amounts. This would be a differentiation of the two alleles by virtue of their quantitative effects by the amount of protein which they make. In our present state of ignorance about the quantitative control of protein synthesis, it is not of course possible to judge the likeliness of Wells and Itano's proposition.

MULTIPLE HEMOGLOBINS

It is a curious fact, discussed earlier in this chapter, that a heterozygote for any of the abnormal hemoglobin genes does not produce hybrid molecules of the type $\alpha_2^A\beta^A\beta^S$. Presumably, each red cell precursor in an A/S individual is itself heterozygous and capable of making β^A and β^S peptide chains. Supporting evidence came recently from the study of a case where four hemoglobin types were present together in one person (Baglioni and Ingram, 1961). Atwater *et al.* (1960) reported that this individual from Philadelphia has the four hemoglobins A, $G_{Philadelphia}$, C, and X. These authors also showed that the C and G abnormalities were inherited in this family independently and that they were nonallelic. Since hemoglobin C was known to be abnormal in the β peptide chain, they proposed that hemoglobin $G_{Philadelphia}$ might be abnormal in the α peptide chain and that hemoglobin X would be abnormal in both the α and the β peptide chains.

Baglioni and Ingram (1961) separated these four components by starch block electrophoresis and fingerprinted them in order to investigate the chemical differences between them. It became immediately apparent that the hemoglobin A and the hemoglobin C components from this individual were of the usual type, but that the hemoglobin G represented a new hemoglobin abnormality (see Figures 3-7, 3-8, 3-9).

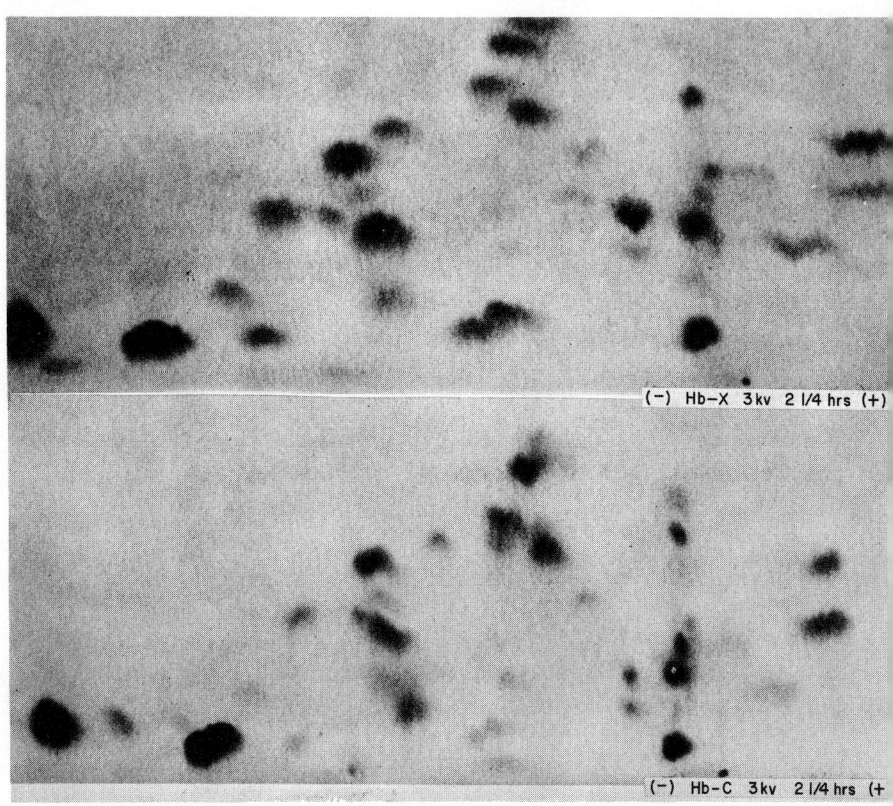

FIGURE 3-7. Photograph of fingerprints of hemoglobins X (above) and C (below)

Electrophoresis, pH 6.4; chromatography, pyridine: isoamyl alcohol: water (35:35:30). (Baglioni and Ingram, 1961.)

It was interesting to see that the four components were present in somewhat similar amounts, hemoglobin A, 35 percent; G, 27 percent; C, 23 percent; and X, 15 percent.

In Figure 3-8 we see tracings of two fingerprints, the top fingerprint is that of normal hemoglobin and the bottom one of hemoglobin

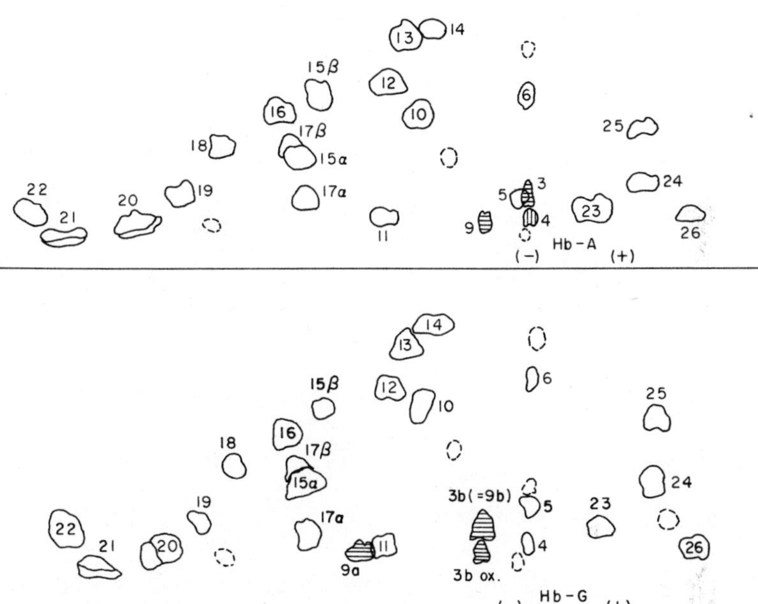

FIGURE 3-8. Tracing of fingerprints of hemoglobins A and $\text{G}_{\text{Philadelphia}}$ Conditions same as Figure 3-7. (Baglioni and Ingram, 1961.)

$\text{G}_{\text{Philadelphia}}$. It turned out that the investigation of the amino acid substitution of this hemoglobin G was not as easy as it had been with sickle-cell hemoglobin. Two peptide spots of hemoglobin A disappear, namely numbers 3 and 9 (see also Table 3-2), and instead three new peptides are visible in the hemoglobin G fingerprint. Strangely enough all this is due to a single amino acid substitution, because peptides 3 and 9 are very closely related, number 9 being equal to number 3 with the addition of an extra lysine residue at the beginning of the peptide

(Figure 3-10). Peptides 3 and 9 are derived from a region of the α peptide chain immediately after a lysyl-lysyl sequence (positions α 60 and α 61) which ought to be completely split into two tryptic peptides plus a free lysine amino acid, but which is in fact only partially split with the formation of additional peptides. These facts are briefly

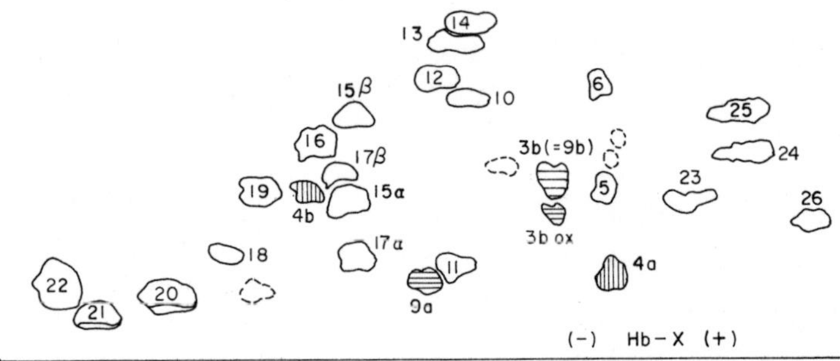

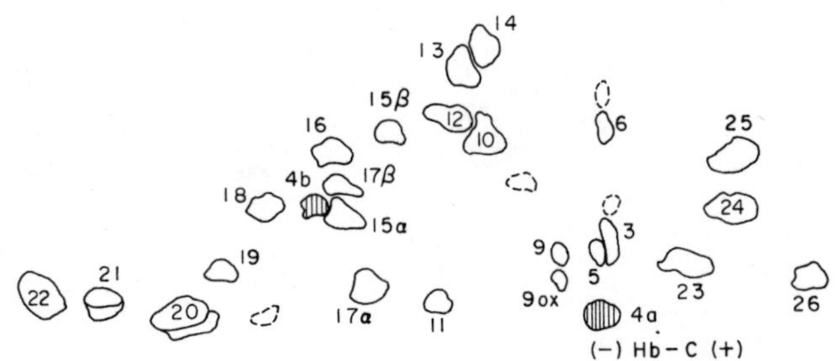

FIGURE 3-9. Tracing of fingerprints of hemoglobins X and C
Conditions same as Figure 3-7. (Baglioni and Ingram, 1961.)

illustrated in Figure 3-10 which shows the relationship between peptides 3 and 9 in the α chain. The lysyl-lysyl sequence already referred to occurs just before the peptide sequence illustrated in the figure. In hemoglobin $G_{\text{Philadelphia}}$ an additional lysine residue occurs replacing asparagine in position α 68. This provides a new point of attack for the hydrolytic action of trypsin and results in the formation of three new peptides in the abnormal hemoglobin. The expected peptide G-3a is not actually clearly resolved in this fingerprint and is not shown in

Figure 3-8. The third peptide visible in that drawing, however, the so-called peptide 3b ox is the oxidized form of the peptide G-3b in which the amino acid methionine is in the sulfoxide form with a consequent change in chromatographic mobility. This extra peptide G-3b ox is therefore to be regarded as an artifact due to the handling of

TABLE 3-2

TRYPTIC PEPTIDES OF THE α AND β CHAINS OF HEMOGLOBIN A

α chain peptides		*β chain peptides*	
*Peptide number**	*Peptide position***	*Peptide number**	*Peptide position***
3	αTp IX	4	βTp I
9	αTp VIII, IX	5	βTp XIII
10	αTp VI	6	βTp IX
11	αTp I, II	12	βTp II
13	αTp V	14	βTp IV
15α	αTp III	15β	βTp XV
16α	αTp XIV	16β	βTp XIV
17α	αTp II	17β	βTp XIV, XV
18	αTp X	19	βTp VI
20α	αTp VII	20β	βTp VII
21α	αTp VII, VIII	21β	βTp VII, VIII
22α	αTp VIII	22β	βTp VIII
23	αTp IV	24	βTp V oxidized***
		25	βTp V
		26	βTp III

* Old numbering system (Ingram, 1958; Baglioni, 1961) as used, for example, in Figures 3-8, 3-9.

** New numbering system (Gerald and Ingram, 1961), based on the known sequence of the tryptic peptides.

*** Peptide 24 is identical with 25, except that the methionine residue is present as its sulfoxide.

the trypsin digest and not an inherent structural feature of the molecule.

The genotype and the phenotype of this individual who produces the four hemoglobins are illustrated in Figure 3-11. One stage of the synthesis of the hemoglobin peptide chains is missing in this drawing, namely the intermediate template RNA or messenger RNA. The structural genes which determine the primary structure of the hemoglobin peptide chain in the usual way are in this individual heterozygous at both the α and the β locus. Each of the four structural genes will send its particular template RNA into the ribosomes of the cell, there

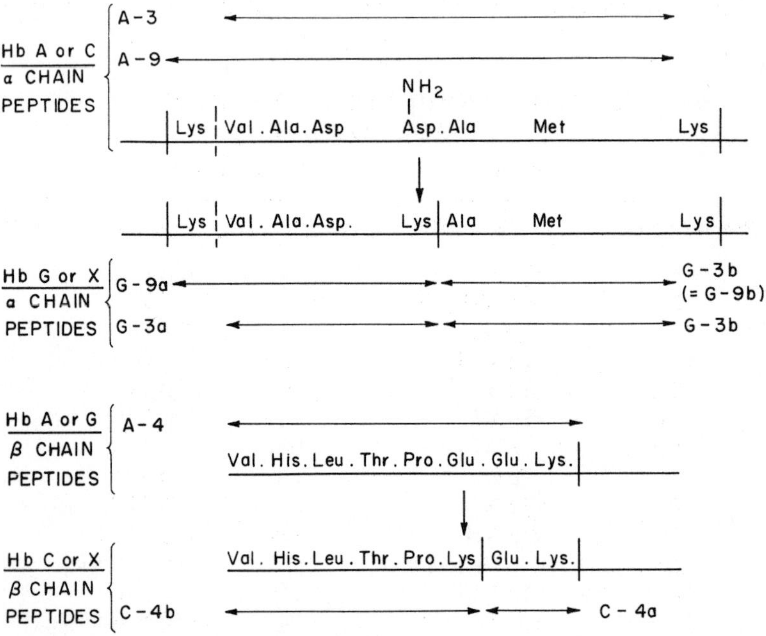

FIGURE 3-10. Diagram of the peptides carrying the abnormalities obtained from hemoglobins A, G, C, X
(Baglioni and Ingram, 1961.)

to synthesize α^A and α^G peptide chains as well as β^A and β^C peptide chains. It appears that these chains are already dimerized before they are liberated into the solution of the cell, so that they are in equilibrium with one another as α_2 or β_2 subunits. These four subunits both normal and abnormal can associate with each other to form the four hemoglobin types, which we recognize.

$$\alpha_2^A + \alpha_2^G + \beta_2^A + \beta_2^C \rightarrow \alpha_2^A\beta_2^A + \alpha_2^G\beta_2^A + \alpha_2^A\beta_2^C + \alpha_2^G\beta_2^C$$

It follows also that a particular ribosome contains only one template RNA molecule which is either normal or abnormal and either α or β; otherwise if those α^A and α^G template RNAs had been present in one and the same ribosome, then we might reasonably have expected to find the formation of truly hybrid hemoglobin molecules of the type $\alpha^A\alpha^G\beta_2^A$, etc. The fact that such hybrids are not found can be taken as evidence for the presence of only a single template per ribosome.

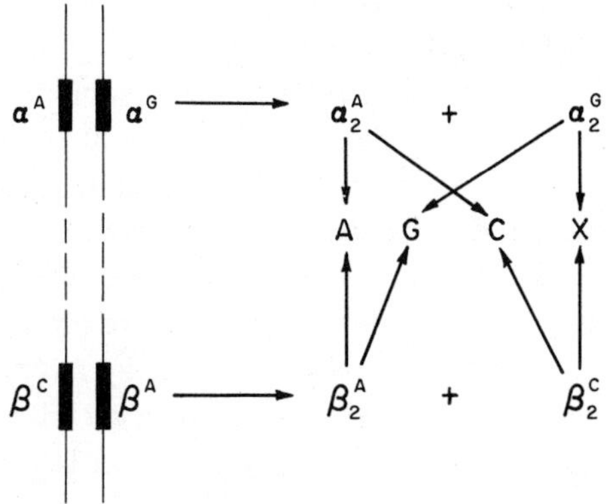

FIGURE 3-11. Genotype (left) and phenotype of the person possessing the four hemoglobins: A, $G_{Philadelphia}$, C, and X
(Courtesy of Dr. C. Baglioni.)

A somewhat similar situation exists in the family described by Smith and Torbert (1958) in which there are individuals having three hemoglobin components: A, Hopkins-2, and S; Hb Ho-2 and S are not alleles. Itano and Robinson (1960) found by dissociation and reassociation studies (Singer and Itano, 1958) that Hopkins-2 is a hemoglobin with an abnormality in the α peptide chain, $\alpha_2^{Ho\text{-}2}\beta_2^A$. Really there are four and not three hemoglobin components in these individuals: Hb A $= \alpha_2^A\beta_2^A$, Hb Hopkins-2 $= \alpha_2^{Ho\text{-}2}\beta_2^A$, Hb S $= \alpha_2^A\beta_2^S$, and Hb Ho-2/S $= \alpha_2^{Ho\text{-}2}\beta_2^S$. Hemoglobin Hopkins-2 is as fast in electrophoresis, as S is slow, compared with hemoglobin A. Therefore, Hb A and Hb Ho-2/S, the doubly abnormal protein, move together in electrophoresis and are not easily distinguished. Cabannes and Portier (1959) have described an individual with three hemoglobin components: Hb A, D, and K, the last being an electrophoretically fast hemoglobin. Perhaps, in this case also the so-called hemoglobin A is really a mixture of normal A and a doubly abnormal hemoglobin in which the effects of the two electrophoretic abnormalities cancel. Such an explanation would suggest that these hemoglobins D and K have abnormalities in different hemoglobin chains and that the genes responsible for them are not allelic. There is however no evidence for either conclusion. Raper *et al.* (1960) reported a family in which mother and daughter have four electrophoretically distinct hemoglobin components: A, $G_{Bristol}$, C, and X (which is the doubly abnormal protein Hb G_{Br}/C). They showed by dissociation experiments that $G_{Bristol}$ is an α chain abnormality, whereas C is the usual β chain variant, so that Hb X may be written as $\alpha_2^{GBr}\beta_2^{C}$. There is strong evidence in this family for non-allelism of the two defects. The genetics is therefore analogous to that in the A, $G_{Philadelphia}$, C, X family described by Atwater *et al.* (1960) and by Baglioni and Ingram (1961). The chemical relationship between hemoglobins $G_{Philadelphia}$ and $G_{Bristol}$ is unknown beyond the fact that both are α chain variants.

HEMOGLOBINS D

We turn now to a discussion of the hemoglobins D (Itano, 1951; Lehmann, 1956), which are characterized (Figure 3-1) by an electrophoretic mobility equal to that of sickle-cell hemoglobin at pH 8.6, but different from S at pH 6 in agar gel (Robinson *et al.*, 1957). In addition, the hemoglobins D do not show the sickling phenomenon nor the disease-producing characteristics of hemoglobin S, although perhaps some forms of hemoglobin D are accompanied by a mild form of hemolytic anemia. Hemoglobin D is found with considerable frequency (between 1 and 2 percent) in some portions of India. Lehmann (1959) estimates the proportion of D carriers to be about 2 percent among Punjabis and 1 percent among Gujeratis. Some years ago Lehmann provided three samples of hemoglobin D, one from a *Turkish* Cypriot (Dα), one from a Gujerati (Dβ) and a third from a Punjabi (Dγ, now called D_{Punjab}). These hemoglobins were purified and subjected to analysis of their tryptic peptides by one-dimensional paper electrophoresis and also by fingerprinting (Benzer *et al.*, 1958). The results of the former technique are illustrated in Figure 3-12. For the purposes of the illustration, the three one-dimensional electrophoreses of the hemoglobin D samples, called D_α, D_β, and D_γ, as well as the comparison digests of hemoglobin A, were cut into thin strips parallel to the direction of electrophoresis. These were then stained with ninhydrin for general peptide material and with specific stains for histidine, arginine, and tyrosine. It may be seen quite clearly that hemoglobin D_α (Turkish Cypriot) is different from the D_β (Gujerati), since they differ from each other and from hemoglobin A by not having a peptide 23 or 26, respectively. Hemoglobin D_γ (Punjabi), on the other hand, appeared almost normal with no visible differences in the peptide pattern, yet the electrophoretic behavior of the parent hemoglobin D_γ was certainly different from the hemoglobin A. In the very bottom line of Figure 3-12, where the peptides are stained for tyrosine, we can see that the digest of hemoglobin D_γ has a greatly reduced tyrosine stain in the neutral band. This was at least a suggestion that an abnormality of hemoglobin D_γ might reside in a tyrosine-containing peptide. However, even without this last piece of evidence, the hemoglobins D_α, D_β, and D_γ are clearly different from each other, since hemoglobin D_γ has both peptides 23 and 26 intact.

These were the first three samples of hemoglobin D which were examined. It was a surprise to find that they all turned out to be different, which was upsetting for those who wish to use the distribution of an abnormal hemoglobin, such as D, for deducing the origins and movements of populations which carry this abnormality. It turns out that the two Indian populations are probably not related with respect to this hemoglobin characteristic, since the mutations which produced D_α and D_β are clearly distinct and separate.

Recently some more samples of hemoglobin D have been examined by Baglioni (1962b). One was the original sample (Benzer *et al.*, 1958) from the Punjab (D_γ), another from a caucasian from North Carolina, one was hemoglobin D_{Chicago} from an Italian family in Chicago (Bowman and Ingram, 1962), the fourth came from Portugal and the

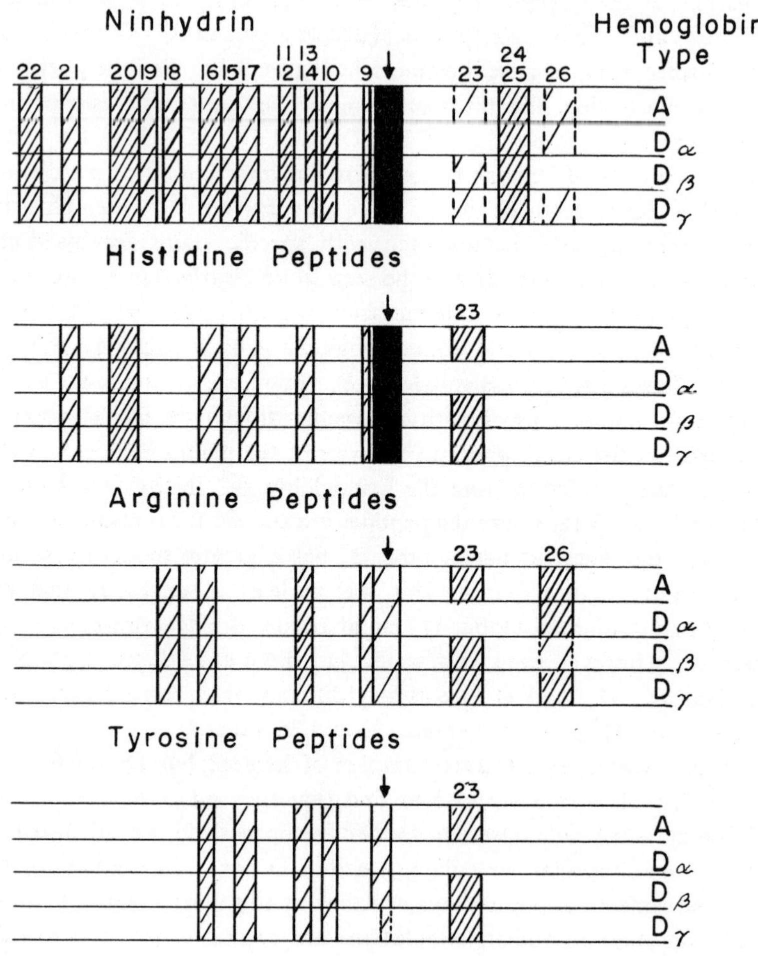

FIGURE 3-12. Comparison by one-dimensional paper electrophoresis at pH 6.4 of tryptic digests of hemoglobins A, D_{α}, D_{β}, and D_{γ} (= D_{Punjab}) (For experimental details, see Benzer *et al.*, 1958.)

fifth from Cyprus from a *Greek* Cypriot. One would naturally expect results similar to those of the first three samples, namely to find differences in hemoglobin structure. Surprisingly, however, this group of hemoglobin D samples all turned out to have identical amino acid substitutions.

In these samples it was necessary to purify the hemoglobin D, since the individuals from which the specimen were obtained were heterozygotes. In Figure 3-13 is shown a typical column chromatographic separation of a hemoglobin A-D mixture; peak 2 is hemoglobin A, and peak 3 hemoglobin D. After concentrations of the two fractions, fingerprints of the tryptic digests showed the patterns reproduced in Figure 3-14, which were identical for all five samples of hemoglobin D. It can be seen that a new peptide, indicated by the arrow, can be found in these hemoglobins D which stains easily for tyrosine. This peptide is derived from an uncharged tyrosine-containing peptide (number 5 or βTp XIII) in the fingerprint of hemoglobin A (Benzer *et al.*, 1958; Bowman and Ingram, 1962), which reacts only weakly with ninhydrin and is therefore hardly visible in the fingerprint. Clearly the fingerprints of these five D's are different from those of the hemoglobin D_α and D_β referred to earlier.

It turns out (Baglioni, 1962b) that in the β chain of these five hemoglobin D samples there is an amino acid substitution in position 121, where glutamine replaces the normally found glutamic acid. This is of course a charge change, since the side chain of glutamic acid is negatively charged and the side chain of glutamine is neutral. Although the abnormal amino acid is only the amide derivative of the normal residue, the substitution is not likely to be an artifact of the method of isolation, since glutamine is thought to be coded for in protein synthesis as a separate amino acid. This change in position 121 of the β chain is far away from the peptide difference previously observed in hemoglobin D_β (somewhere in the region β 18 – 30) or indeed from that of hemoglobin D_α which is moreover in the α peptide chain.

We have here a curious situation of seven hemoglobin D samples from widely different geographical localities. Of these, five appear to be identical in spite of their widely scattered origin; the other two are

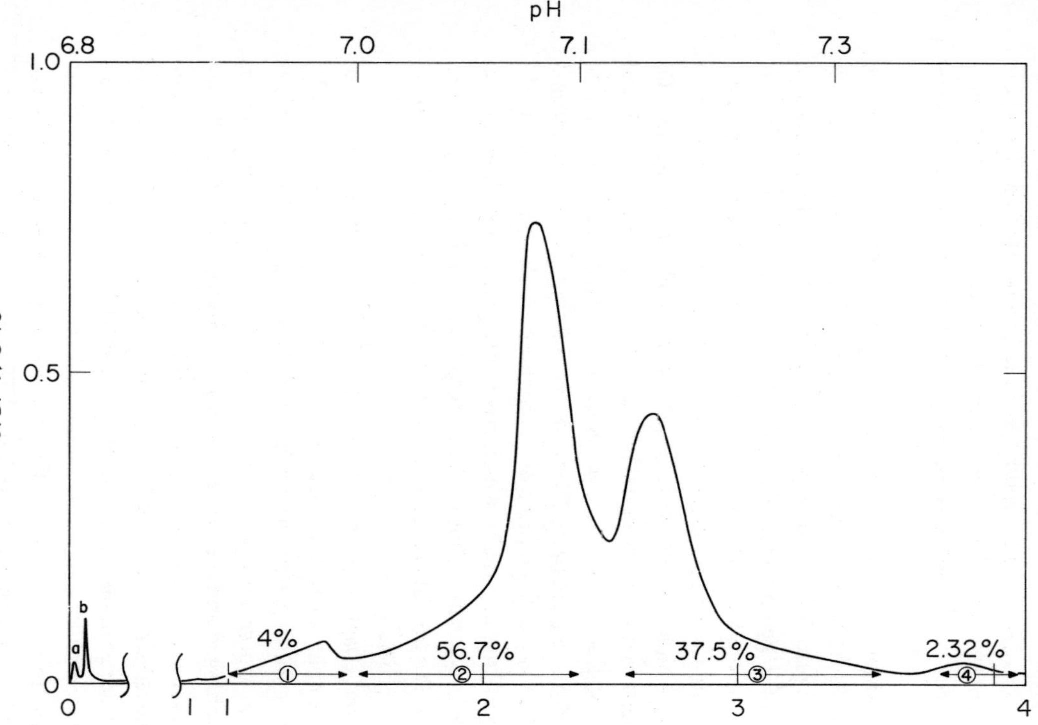

FIGURE 3-13. Separation of hemoglobins A and D_{Punjab} from blood of a heterozygote by column chromatography
(For details, see Baglioni, 1962.)

different from each other and from the group of five. We do not know whether the three different chemical types observed are due to only three mutational events or whether on the other hand the five identical hemoglobin D samples are really derived from one and the same mutation which was spread by the movement of individuals. One is inclined to favor the last possibility, because the hemoglobin D sample

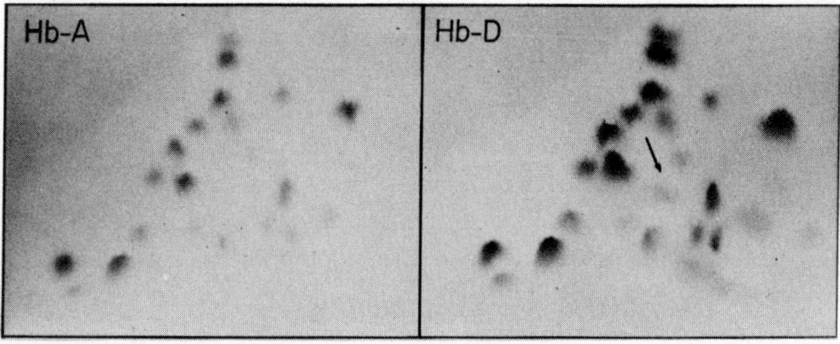

FIGURE 3-14. Photographs of fingerprints of hemoglobins A and D_{Punjab}
(Baglioni, 1962.)

from the Punjab came from a population where this abnormality reaches a frequency of 1.8 percent; whereas the hemoglobin D collected in this country from North Carolina, Chicago, and that from Portugal occur only very rarely. In other words, since a very large number of individuals possess this gene, it is easy to see how migration of a few would give rise to isolated families scattered throughout the world. Perhaps the "passing stranger" of human genetics was in these instances a Punjabi! An alternative view would suggest that the mutation leading to the glutamic acid to glutamine change in position β 121 has arisen more than once. Is this mutation site a "hot" spot?

HEMOGLOBINS M

Hemoglobin M was historically the first abnormal hemoglobin to be described in a rare hereditary methemoglobinemia (Hörlein and Weber 1948; Gerald, 1960). It turns out that in this disease two of the iron atoms of some of the hemoglobin molecules are in the oxidized (methemoglobin) state instead of being in the usual reduced state. Moreover, this methemoglobin has an abnormal absorption spectrum. Such a methemoglobin derivative of hemoglobin is incapable of combining with molecular oxygen and therefore cannot carry out its normal physiological role, leading to clinical symptoms of cyanosis. More recently a number of instances of this rare disease have been discovered (see in Gerald, 1960; Gerald and Efron, 1961), some in this country and one in Japan in addition to the original German type. Of these, hemoglobin M_{Boston}, hemoglobin $M_{Saskatoon}$, and hemoglobin $M_{Milwaukee\ 1}$ were analyzed by Gerald and Efron (1961). It turns out that the individuals with these conditions are all heterozygotes who have a mixture of hemoglobin A and the particular hemoglobin M in their blood.

Tryptic digests of the purified hemoglobin M were subjected to fingerprinting and other types of examination by Gerald and Efron. They found the abnormalities of these hemoglobins M to reside in specific single amino acid substitutions which are illustrated in Figures 3-15 and 3-16. On the left of Figure 3-15 is shown a small portion of the α peptide chain of hemoglobin A in diagrammatic form, beginning with residue 55 and going on to residue 64; the whole chain is 141 residues long. If we may transfer the details of protein structure discovered by Kendrew in the related protein myoglobin from the sperm whale, we would find that the stretch of amino acid sequence shown in Figure 3-15 is in the form of an α helix and that near this α helix is the iron atom of the heme group (see Figure 2-4). This iron atom is usually bonded to the imidazole side chain of a histidine residue of the α chain, which is not shown in the Figure 3-15, since it belongs to a different portion of the α peptide chain. The histidine residue which is shown is on the side of the iron atom opposite to the "bonding" histidine residue. Of the six coordination positions of the iron atom four are occupied by the four nitrogen atoms of the porphyrin ring of the heme group, a fifth is coordinated to the "bonding" histidine residue already mentioned, and the sixth position is free and available for the reversible combination with oxygen molecules or the other ligands, such as carbon monoxide or water. However, this sixth

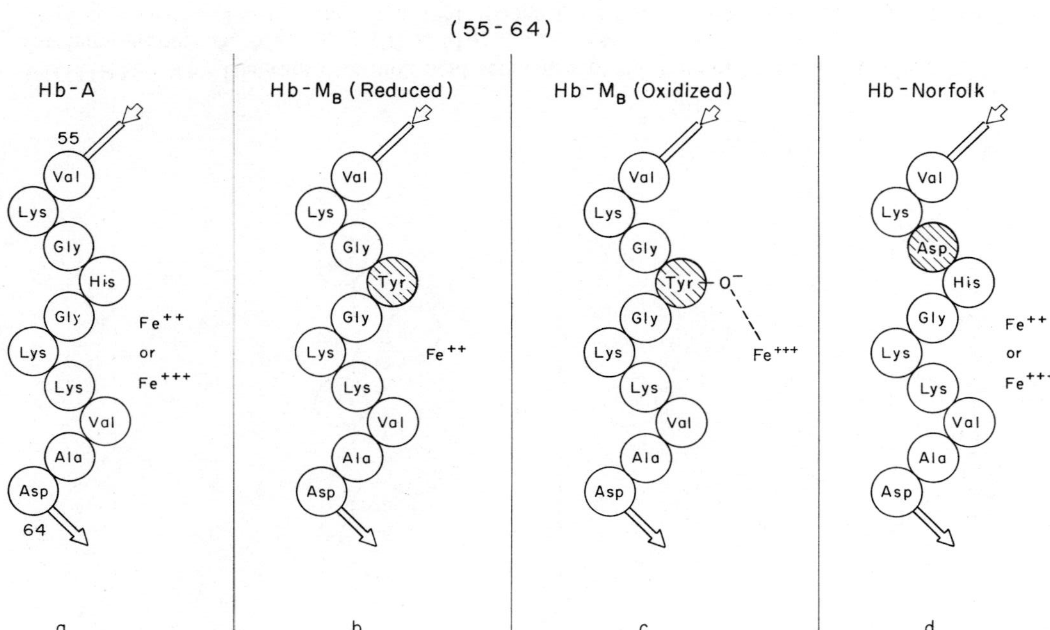

FIGURE 3-15. Diagram of amino acid sequences of the human α chain near the heme group for hemoglobins A, M_{Boston} (Hb-Ma), and Norfolk

Prepared from data of Gerald and Efron, 1961, and Baglioni, 1961. (Courtesy of Dr. C. Baglioni.)

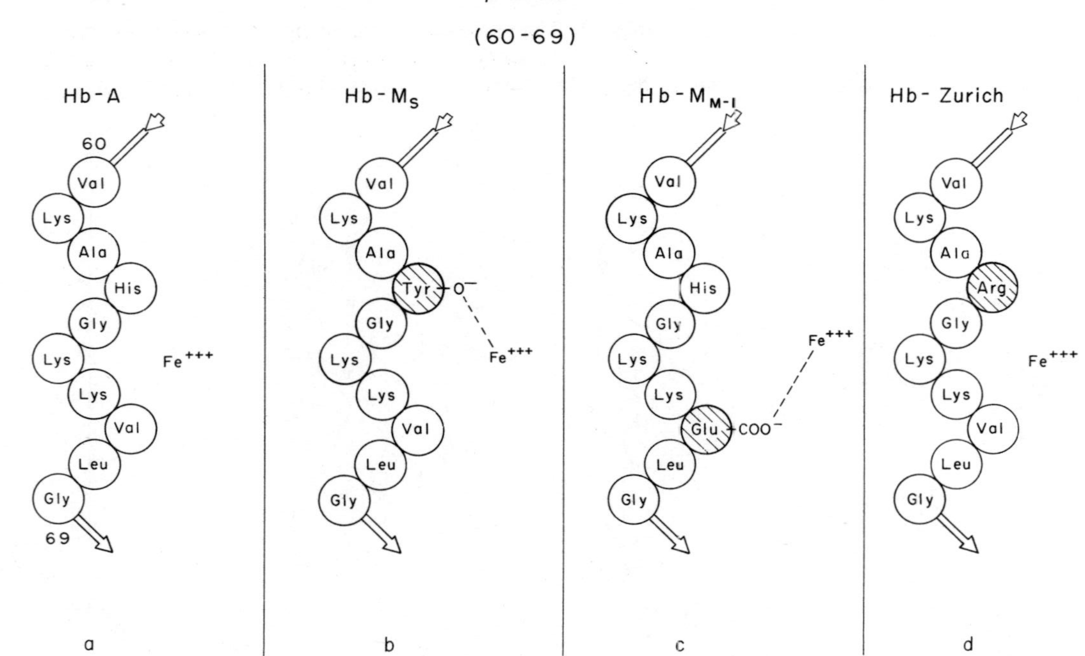

FIGURE 3-16. Diagram of amino acid sequences of the human β chain near the heme group for hemoglobins A, $M_{Saskatoon}$ (M_S), $M_{Milwaukee-1}$ (M_{M-1}), and Zürich
Prepared from data of Gerald and Efron, 1961; Kingma and Muller, 1961. (Courtesy of Dr. C. Baglioni.)

coordination position points straight at the histidine residue illustrated in Figure 3-15.

In hemoglobin M_{Boston} there is an amino acid substitution in the α peptide chain such that the histidine residue in position 58 is replaced by tyrosine. Nothing much happens as the result of the substitution so long as the iron atom remains in the ferrous state. As soon, however, as it becomes oxidized to ferric iron, and this happens to a small extent spontaneously, the neighboring phenol side chain of the tyrosine residue is in just the right position to bond to the ferric iron as a phenolate complex. This is a very stable complex, so much so that the enzymes normally present in the red cell, whose job it is to keep the iron reduced, cannot reduce the phenolate complex. Therefore half the molecule of hemoglobin M_{Boston}, namely the two α chains, remains in the methemoglobin form and is therefore incapable of combining with oxygen. On the other hand, the iron atoms of the β chains of this hemoglobin M are presumably normal or approximately normal and we would expect them to remain active.

HEMOGLOBINS NORFOLK AND M

There is a mutation of adult hemoglobin known as hemoglobin Norfolk which was discovered by Ager, Lehmann, and Vella (1958) in Norfolk, England. The amino acid substitution which characterizes this particular abnormality has been worked out by Baglioni (1962a). He found that the glycine residue in position 57 in the normal α peptide chain has been replaced by aspartic acid in hemoglobin Norfolk. This is in the position next to the histidine which suffers replacement by tyrosine in hemoglobin M_{Boston}. However, in contrast to hemoglobin M_{Boston}, the spectrum and reactivity of the heme group is unaffected by this amino acid substitution in hemoglobin Norfolk. So far as we can tell, hemoglobin Norfolk, a rare mutant, does not show any physiological abnormality. This is especially strange in view of the fact that another mutant having a new carboxyl side chain near the iron atom (Hb $M_{Milwaukee\ 1}$) does form a strong, abnormal ferric complex; yet in hemoglobin Norfolk, the carboxyl side chain of the new aspartic acid residue is apparently not in the right position to form a complex.

HEMOGLOBINS M AND ZURICH

In Figure 3-16 we see the corresponding section of the β peptide chain of hemoglobin A from position 60 to 69. Again this is a helical region close to the iron atom of the heme group of the β chain. As previously, the 6th coordinating position of this iron atom which normally combines with oxygen points in the direction of a histidine residue in position 63. In hemoglobin $M_{Saskatoon}$ Gerald and Efron (1961) were also able to demonstrate a substitution of this particular histidine residue by tyrosine. Again, the new tyrosine residue is in the right position to complex with the oxidized form of the iron atom of the heme group. A stable complex results which is difficult to reduce and hence a persistent methemoglobin of the β chain results.

The third hemoglobin M ($M_{Milwaukee\ 1}$) which we will discuss here, also forms a stable complex between the ferric iron of the β chain heme group and the side chain of an abnormal amino acid. This time, however, the abnormality resides in position β 67 (Gerald and Efron, 1961) and consists of a replacement of a valine residue by glutamic acid. As it happens, this is the reverse of the amino acid substitution in sickle cell hemoglobin, but this fact does not appear to have any particular importance. The new glutamic acid residue is just four residues away from position β 63 where the tyrosine side chain was sterically capable of complexing with the heme iron. Four residues away on an α helix means roughly one turn of the helix; that is to say, two amino acids separated in sequence by three residues will have side chains pointing in the same direction. It is not surprising therefore that glutamic acid can complex with its ionized carboxylate group at the end of its side chain to the iron atom of the heme group. This stable complex, like the others, leads to the abnormal methemoglobin and to the symptoms of the hemoglobin M disease.

Another rare hemoglobin abnormality which is close to the hemoglobins M, namely hemoglobin Zürich, was analyzed by Muller and Kingma (1961). They found a new arginine residue which had taken the place of the normal histidine in position 63 of the β peptide chain. Although this is the same position as that occupied by the abnormal tyrosine in hemoglobin $M_{Saskatoon}$, there seems to be no evidence for any complex formation of the arginine side chain with the iron atom of the heme group. Consequently, the possession of this hemoglobin Zürich abnormality is not to be considered as being deleterious like a hemoglobin M type abnormality. On the other hand, there are reports that hemoglobin Zürich inside the red cells will precipitate under certain conditions, but the clinical significance of this finding is not yet clear. The three-dimensional aspect of the ability of the hemoglobin M amino acid substitutions to complex with the iron atom of the heme group can be most clearly seen in Figure 2-4 where in Kendrew's model of the myoglobin molecule the coordination positions of the iron atom are quite clearly visible. The relationship to the iron atom of a tyrosine residue and of a glutamic acid residue in positions β 63 and β 67, respectively, can also be easily envisaged.

SUMMARY OF ABNORMALITIES

Figure 3-17 shows the summary of the chemical abnormalities in a variety of human hemoglobins known at the time of writing. This picture is a composite of the work done in a number of laboratories; it also relies to a large extent on the chemical information obtained from the total amino acid sequence of the α and β peptide chains illustrated in an earlier chapter. Clearly, the various amino acid substitutions are distributed along the α and β peptide chains and they do not seem to be confined to any particular region of the peptide chain. There are, at the moment, more abnormalities in the first half of each chain, but it is doubtful whether this unequal distribution is statistically significant. On the other hand we would certainly not expect that any amino acid whatsoever in the peptide chains could be substituted without impunity, that is without affecting the physiological function of the molecule. Surely there would be some, such as the heme-linked histidine residue or those of Braunitzer's so-called "basic center" (α 56 – 61, β 61 – 66 in Figure 2-5) for which an amino acid substitution will be "forbidden."

There are three points along the β chain where we seem to get more than one amino acid substitution—in positions 6, 63, and 121. The data is still too meager to substantiate the suggestion that these might represent favored mutational sites, but as more data accumulate this point might become a little clearer. It is beginning to look, as if there are more mutations to be found in the β peptide chain than there are

α Chain

	1	2	16	30	57	58	68	116	141
			+	−		+		−	+
	Val.	Leu....	Lys....	Glu....	Gly.	His....	Asp. NH_2.......	Glu	Arg
Hb I			− .Asp.						
Hb $G_{Honolulu}$				.Glu. NH_2.					
Hb Norfolk					− .Asp.				
Hb M_{Boston}						.Tyr.			
Hb $G_{Philadelphia}$							+ .Lys.		
Hb $O_{Indonesia}$								+ .Lys.	

β Chain

	1	2	3	6	7	26	63	67	121	146
		+		−	−	−	+		−	+
	Val.	His.	Leu....	Glu.	Glu....	Glu....	His....	Val.	Glu.......	His
Hb S				.Val.						
Hb C				+ .Lys.						
Hb $G_{San\ José}$					.Gly.					
Hb E						+ .Lys.				
Hb $M_{Saskatoon}$							.Tyr.			
Hb $M_{Milwaukee}$								− .Glu.		
Hb D_{Punjab} (= D_γ)									.Glu. NH_2.	
Hb Zürich							+ .Arg.			
Hb O_{Arabia}									+ .Lys.	

Abnormal Human Hemoglobins

FIGURE 3-17. Diagrammatic summary of the known abnormalities of human hemoglobin

in the α chain. Again, it is not clear whether this difference is statistically significant, since the numbers involved are still quite small.

It is, however, interesting to see that the handful of hemoglobins which are found with high frequency are all in the β chain. These are hemoglobin S, C, E, and D_{Punjab}. All the others with the possible exception of $G_{Philadelphia}$ are rare or very rare. This is not surprising when we consider that the β peptide chain contributes only to the formation of the adult hemoglobin, whereas the α peptide chain is a part of both the adult and the fetal hemoglobin, as well as of hemoglobin A_2. Therefore, we might imagine that an alteration in the α chain would be more deleterious, since it would affect both fetal and adult hemoglobin. The fetus is a more sensitive organism and a deleterious mutation in the α peptide chain (see Lie-Enjo, 1961) will not allow compensation by increased production of one of the other hemoglobin types, such as fetal hemoglobin or hemoglobin A_2. An alteration in the α peptide chain is therefore more drastic. On the other hand, abnormalities in the β peptide chain can, and to some extent are, compensated for by the formation of fetal hemoglobin. The fetus in the case of a β chain abnormality is largely protected, since its fetal hemoglobin will be normal. In addition, and especially in the first few years of life, some benefit will be derived after birth through an ability to make some normal hemoglobin F. For these reasons we are not surprised to find that the abnormalities which occur with high frequencies are confined to the β chain.

Finally it should be noted that the abnormalities listed in Figure 3-17 are, of course, all electrophoretic mutants, because this is how they are first picked up. Since electrophoresis is such a simple technique, thousands of people have been screened for electrophoretic hemoglobin mutants. However, one can also claim that a change in the hemoglobin molecule involving a difference in the charge of that molecule might have a more profound physiological effect on the functioning of the molecule hemoglobin, than would a change which does not alter charged amino acids. Presumably it is a combination of these factors that contributes to the picture which we actually see. In Figure 3-18 is a more fanciful way of illustrating the positions of the amino acid exchanges in hemoglobin. The symmetry of the molecule is clearly portrayed.

THE ABNORMAL HEMOGLOBINS AND THE GENETIC CODE

Smith (1962) has recently published his interpretation of the amino acid changes in the human hemoglobins in terms of the so-called code

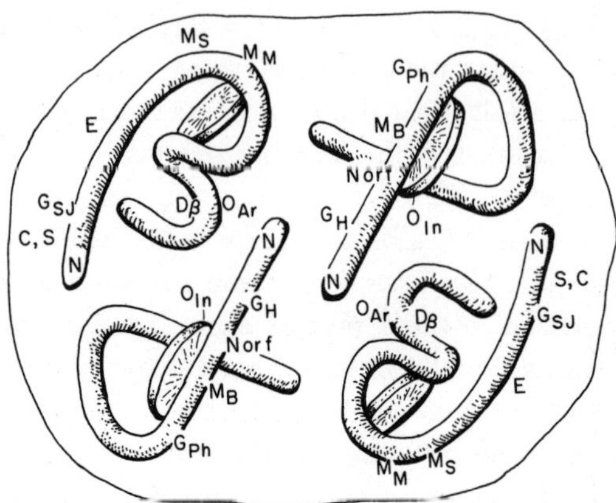

FIGURE 3-18. Diagram showing the location of the abnormalities of human hemoglobin in the idealized structure of the molecule

letters of protein biosynthesis (Matthaei *et al.*, 1962; Speyer *et al.*, 1962). Assuming, for the time being, that the code controlling the synthesis of hemoglobin is a triplet code (Crick *et al.*, 1961), analogous or identical to the one assumed to exist in the bacterial system, we can see in Figure 3-19, taken from Smith's article, that all the known amino acid exchanges in the hemoglobins can be explained in terms of single base changes in the corresponding code letters. It should be

	Hemoglobin Type	Code Letters
Glu → Val	S	UAG → UUG
Glu → Lys	C, E, O	UAG → UAA
Glu → Gly	$G_{San\ José}$	UAG → UGG
Glu → Glu. N	$G_{Honolulu}$, D_{Punjab}	UAG → UCG
Val → Glu	$M_{Milwaukee-I}$	UUG → UAG
Asp → Lys	G_{Phila}	UGA → UAA
Gly → Asp	Norfolk	UGG → UGA
Lys → Asp	I	UAA → UGA
His → Tyr	M_{Boston}, $M_{Saskatoon}$	UAC → UAU
His → Arg	Zürich	UAC → UGC

FIGURE 3-19. The triplet code letters and the amino acid substitutions in the abnormal human hemoglobins (After Smith, 1962.)

pointed out that the code actually given is that assumed to exist on the template RNA and that strictly speaking the corresponding DNA code would be the reciprocal of the codes given; for example UAG in the template RNA would really be ATC in the coding strand of DNA. However, the argument remains the same, since in either case Smith can explain the observed amino acid changes on the basis of altering only a single base in the code. Of course, this is the minimum change, and a more extensive alteration to produce the amino acid exchanges is also conceivable. Nevertheless, it is satisfying to be able to give such a simple explanation for the mutations observed in this system. We need to assume for this argument, however, that the hemoglobin mutants have arisen as single mutational events; really this is only an assumption, for which we have no proof.

It is also noteworthy that the amino acid differences which Stretton found between the β chain of hemoglobin A and the δ chain of hemoglobin A_2 (Ingram and Stretton, 1961) are also all accounted for by single base alterations in the corresponding code letters (Smith, 1962). Here we have even less assurance that the observed alterations are the result of single mutational events rather than the result of a series of steps.

Hemoglobin is, of course, only one example of a protein which carries this type of mutational change. There are now several microbiological systems known in which this kind of mutation has been observed. We can mention particularly the alkaline phosphatase system of *E. coli* which is being studied by Garen, Levinthal, and Rothman (1961). Of particular interest are the induced mutational alterations in tobacco mosaic virus which have been so brilliantly investigated recently by Wittmann in Tübingen (1961) and by Tsugita and Fraenkel-Conrat in Berkeley (1962). They have a great many mutants now as the result of treating the infectious RNA of this virus with the chemical mutagen nitrous acid. The mutants show a spectrum of single amino acid substitutions scattered throughout the molecule. Nearly all of them may be explained in terms of single base alterations in the Nirenberg-Ochoa coding system. It should also be noted that in this particular case RNA is itself the genetic material in contrast to the human system.

Perhaps it also serves as messenger RNA. Not all of the Wittmann mutants can be explained in such a simple manner and it is believed that those which cannot be so explained are the result of spontaneous mutations which would not necessarily have to follow the chemical course anticipated for nitrous acid.

MUTATIONAL EFFECTS IN TRYPTOPHAN SYNTHETASE

Another enzyme of the bacterium *E. coli* has been studied by Yanofsky's group (Helinski and Yanofsky, 1962). Mutants obtained by treatment of the bacterium with ultraviolet light produce a particular protein, a portion of the so-called A protein of tryptophane synthetase which is defective. Yanofsky has obtained a whole series of mutants of which one is particularly interesting, the so-called mutant A-46. Here there is an amino acid substitution where glycine is replaced by glutamic acid. At this stage the precise position of this glycine residue in the peptide chain of this A protein is not known. Another mutant, A-23, is clearly very close to A-46. It turns out that the same glycine amino acid residue has been replaced by arginine. Altogether there are some nine mutants of the A-protein which are located in this area of the peptide chain. Of these the two mutants affecting the same glycine residue are extremely close together with a recombination frequency of about 0.004 percent. Since the recombination length of the whole A chain is 2.5 percent and since Yanofsky knows that there are some 280 amino acid residues in that chain, it follows that mutant A-46 and A-23 are likely to be located within the same coding unit. This is a most interesting result, although one cannot yet calculate with any degree of confidence the length of the coding unit merely because the measurement of the recombination frequency as low as 0.004 percent is technically very difficult.

HIDDEN MUTATIONS

Now we must turn to a totally different problem: How many "hidden" mutations will we find among the hemoglobins of a normal populations of people, and how constant is the chemical composition of such a "normal" protein in the population? We find there are no data as yet in the literature to answer these questions. Recently (Ingram, unpublished) a survey of the chemical structure of samples of normal hemoglobin from individuals has been carried out at M.I.T. at the suggestion of Dr. J. V. Neel in an attempt to answer these questions. Samples ($n = 120$) were taken mostly from Caucasians, but including also four Chinese, one Indian, one Arab, and one Burmese. The samples were examined by electrophoresis in which all were found to be identical. On examination of each hemoglobin sample by fingerprinting (Ingram, 1958) and by an examination of the tryptic peptides by specific staining for particular amino acids (Benzer *et al.*, 1958), no abnormalities could be detected. These tests cover some 30 percent of the hemoglobin molecule. In addition, three large tryptic peptides from each hemoglobin sample were isolated and analyzed quantitatively in the Moore and Stein automatic amino acid analyzer—another 15 percent of each molecule, making a total of 45 percent. Within the technical limitations of the method no abnormality was found, but then it must be remembered that in the quantitative amino acid analysis under our conditions some 20 percent of the samples were outside of one quarter of an amino acid residue from the mean value of that residue for all 120 samples. Had there been a hidden mutation in one of the hemoglobin samples resulting in an amino acid exchange, such an individual would have been almost certainly a heterozygote. Therefore the loss or gain of the affected amino acid in one of the peptides would have been at most one half of a residue. No changes as large as that were observed, but since the standard error for some of the amino acids were as high as 0.4 (they range mostly 0.1–0.25) of an amino acid residue, we cannot exclude the possibility that some of the samples which had a small deviation from the mean might have been a hidden mutation. All we can do in this case is to set a limit on the probability of finding a hidden mutation and to state that the probability is not very large, since at least 80 percent of the samples were seen to be normal within our limits.

4

THE QUANTITATIVE CONTROL OF PROTEIN SYNTHESIS: HEMOGLOBIN A_2

In a normal adult there is a minor electrophoretic component, hemoglobin A_2, amounting to about 2.5 percent of the total hemoglobin (Kunkel and Wallenius, 1955). This is always present, although in some diseases such as β chain thalassemia the proportion may rise, rarely exceeding 7 or 8 percent. The starch block electrophoresis of various types of hemoglobin may be seen in Figure 4-1. The sample labeled "Normal" shows clearly the major hemoglobin component A_1 ($\alpha_2^A\beta_2^A$). Behind it may be seen hemoglobin A_2 which we can write as $\alpha_2^A\delta_2^{A_2}$. In front of the major hemoglobin component is the so-called hemoglobin A_3 which is a derivative of hemoglobin A_1 found in old cells. Muller (1961) has shown that this hemoglobin A_3 contains glutathione bound firmly to the hemoglobin molecule and clearly visible in fingerprints of hemoglobin A_3. It is not known just how glutathione is bound to hemoglobin A_3, how many equivalents of this peptide are contained in the molecule and whether there are perhaps other changes as well. Possibly glutathione which is very abundant inside the red cells eventually gets bound to hemoglobin via a disulfide linkage and is liberated in the course of tryptic digestion by a process of disulfide interchange.

The proportion of hemoglobin A_2 is remarkably constant in normal people. Recently Stretton (Stretton and Ingram, 1961) has analyzed

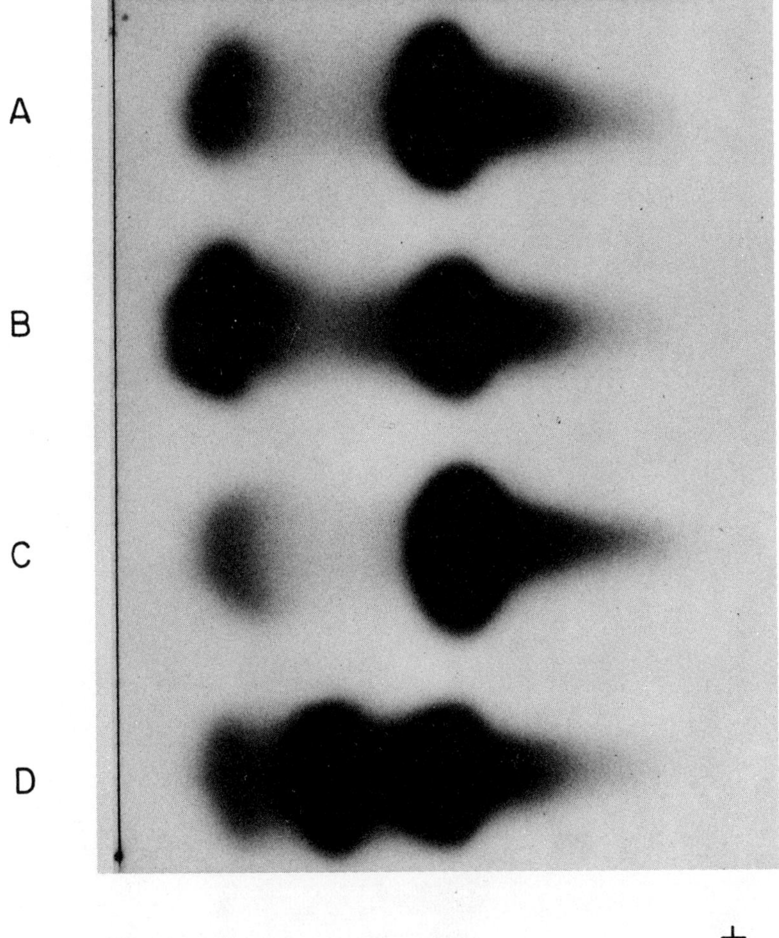

FIGURE 4-1. Starch block electrophoretic patterns of cyanmethemoglobins in veronal buffer (pH 8.6, ionic strength 0.05) for 22 hours (Courtesy of Dr. P. S. Gerald.)

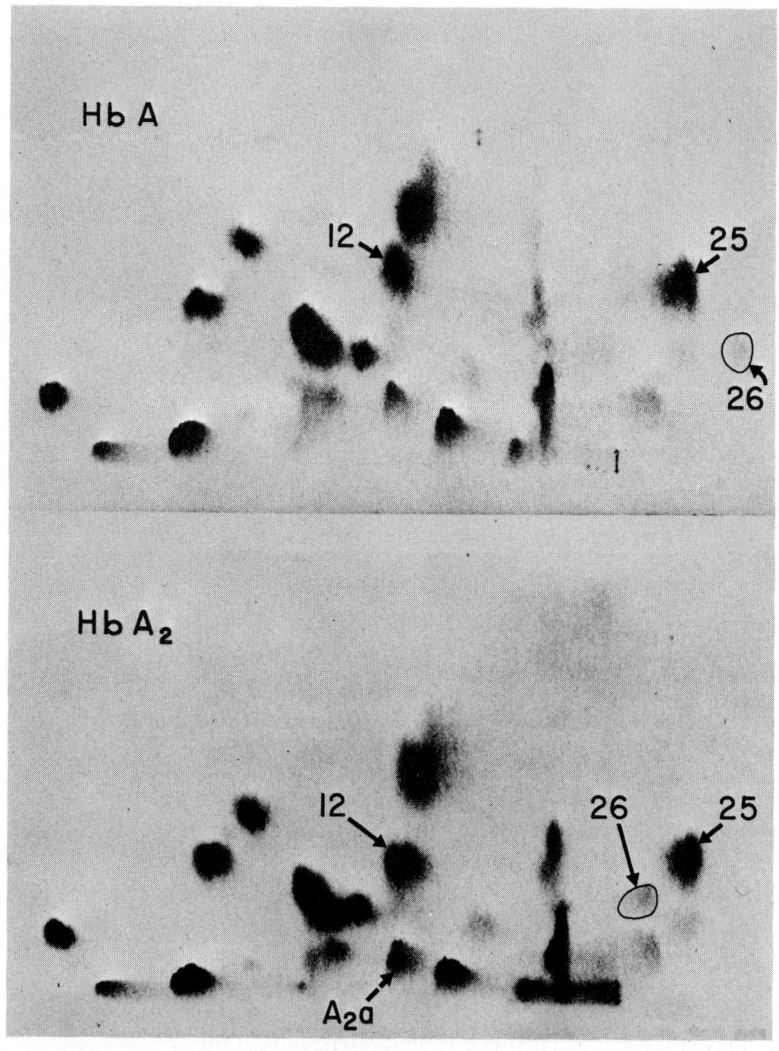

FIGURE 4-2. Photographs of fingerprints of tryptic digests of hemoglobin A and A_2, at pH 6.6 and in n-butanol: acetic acid: water (3:1:1) Peptides 26 from Hb-A and Hb-A_2 are outlined; peptides 12, 25 and A_2 are indicated. (Ingram and Stretton, 1961.)

purified hemoglobin A_2 by fingerprinting. Examples are shown in Figure 4-2 where the bottom portion is that of hemoglobin A_2 with some of the known chemical changes indicated—peptides 12, 25, 26, and A_2a. All the differences between hemoglobin A and hemoglobin A_2 so far detected are located in the δ peptide chain of hemoglobin A_2 (Figure 4-3) giving rise to the conviction that hemoglobin A and A_2 contain the same α peptide chains.

The so-called peptide 12 (corresponding to peptide βTp II in the β chain) assumed a new and lower position in chromatography in fingerprints of hemoglobin A_2. Stretton found that there are two amino acid changes in this peptide, that a serine is replaced by threonine and that a threonine is replaced by asparagine. Both these are exchanges involving uncharged amino acids and therefore the electrophoretic position of peptide 12 remains unaltered. It speaks for the power of the fingerprinting method that it is able to pick up the rather subtle differences in chemical constitution involved in these alterations. On the other hand peptide 25 (corresponding to peptide βTp V in the β chain) does not show any unusual behavior in these fingerprints. However, a more careful comparison of all peptides in an extended chromatographic run (Ingram, 1961b, p. 97 – 98) did reveal an alteration in mobility. This was eventually traced by Stretton to a replacement of threonine by serine in position 50 of the δ peptide chain. It is not surprising that the loss of a methyl group in a nonadecapeptide did not show in the fingerprint, but it is remarkable that it showed up at all in chromatography. Peptide 26 (corresponding to peptide βTp III in the β chain) assumes a very different electrophoretic position in these fingerprints, due to the loss of a negative charge through the replacement of a glutamic acid residue by the uncharged amino acid alanine. This exchange accounts for only half of the electrophoretic difference between hemoglobin A_1 and hemoglobin A_2. It may be that the other electrophoretic difference between the two proteins resides in the so-called peptide A_2a which is indicated in Figure 4-2. This represents a new peptide for which there is no counterpart in the normal fingerprint pattern of hemoglobin A. We should note, however, at this point that a normal fingerprint of tryptic peptides represents

The β and δ Peptide Chains of

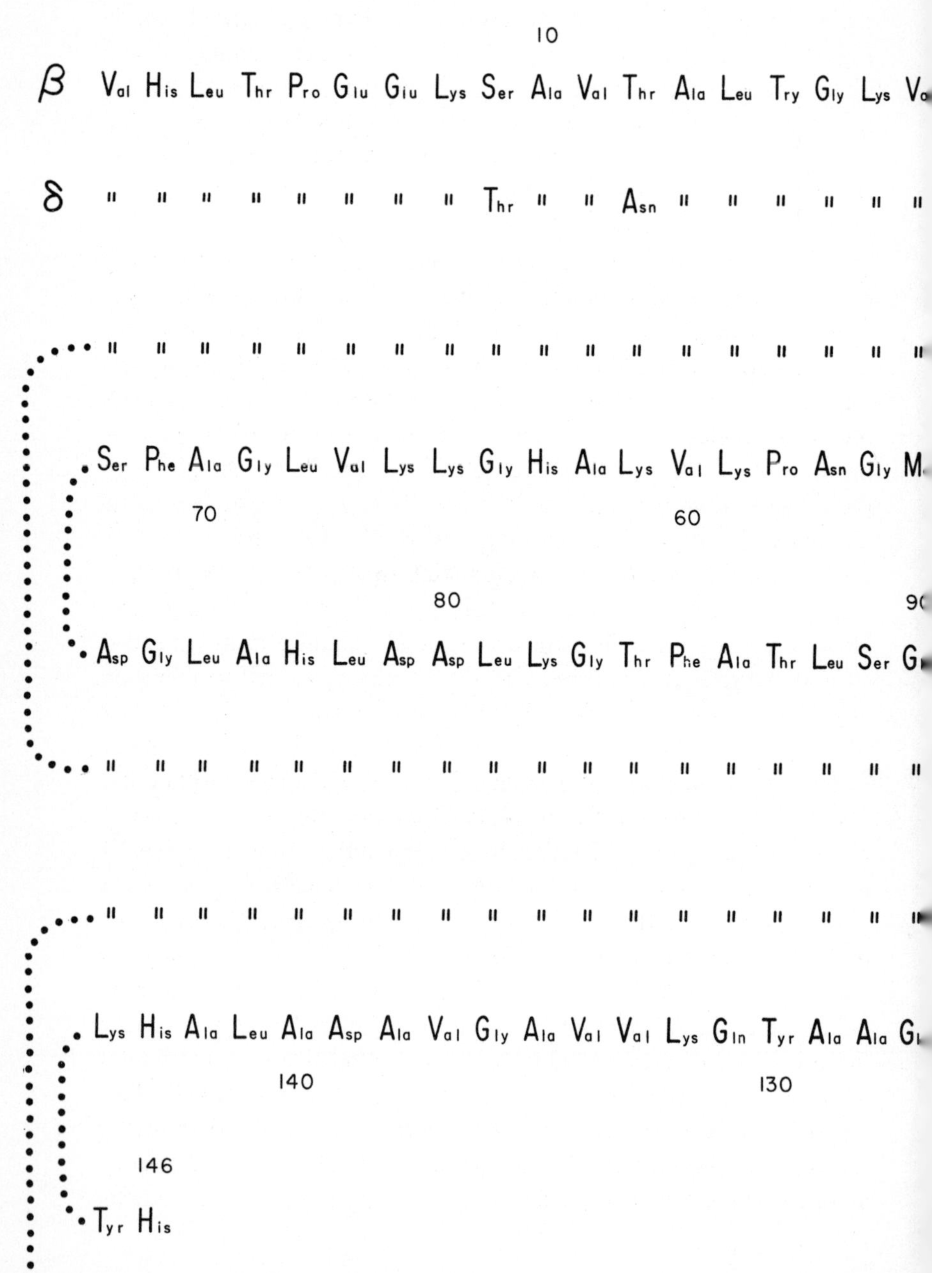

the Human Hemoglobins A and A_2

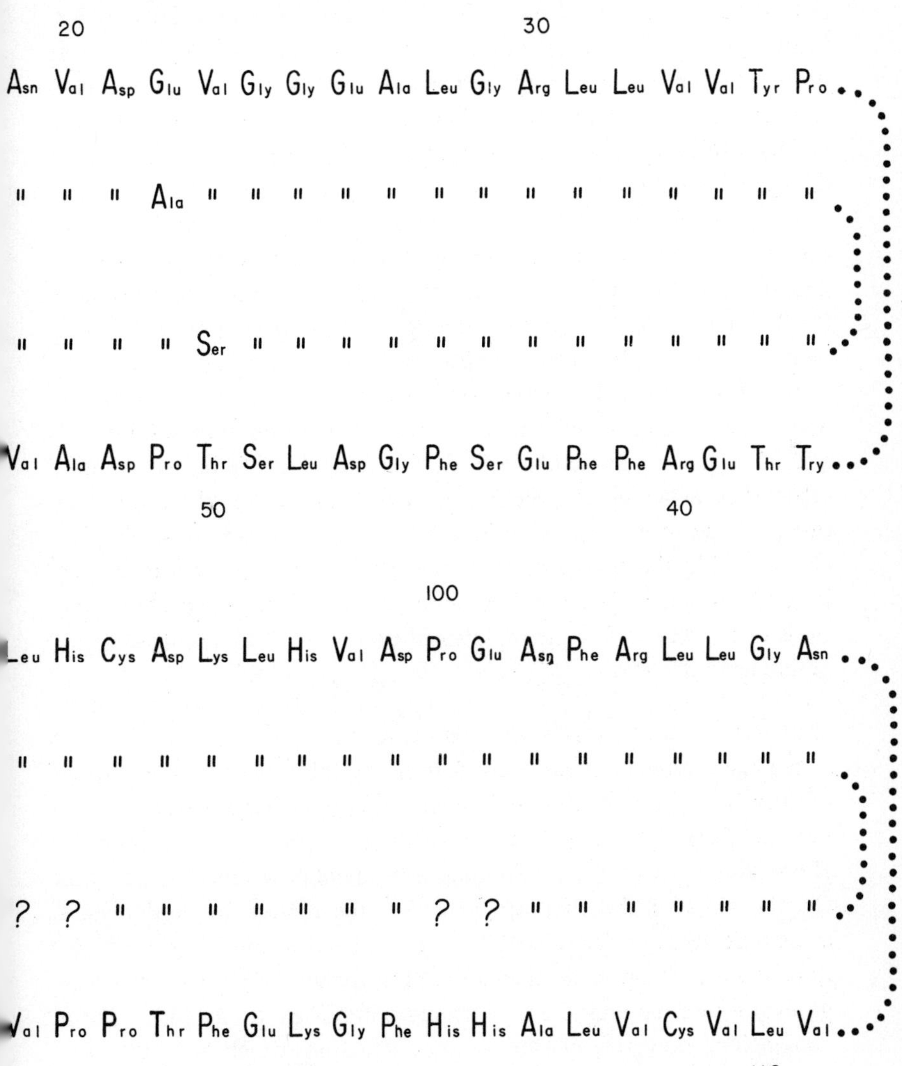

FIGURE 4-3. Diagram of the amino acid sequence of the human β and δ chains

The δ chain sequence is not yet fully determined; portions where an amino acid substitution is suspected are indicated by ? (After Ingram and Stretton, 1961, 1962a, b.)

only about two thirds of the molecule, because the remainder remains insoluble as the so-called core. It may well be that A_2a becomes liberated from the core by the introduction of a new lysine or arginine residue into the molecule, possibly in the position corresponding to residue 116 of the β chain. Stretton finds that peptide A_2a is a small tetrapeptide containing the amino acids asparagine, phenylalanine, glycine, and lysine (formula: Asp.NH_2.Phe.Gly.Lys). It is likely that the total number of amino acid exchanges which distinguish the δ peptide chain from the β peptide chain may rise to some 7 or 8 residues (Figure 4-3). The rest of the peptides appear to be similar in both peptide chains with respect to their amino acid composition at least. It remains to be seen whether or not they contain inversions of the amino acid sequence such as is observed for example in residues 21 and 22 of the γ peptide chain of fetal hemoglobin compared to the β chain (Schroeder *et al.*, 1962). In addition it seems likely that the order of the tryptic peptides is identical in the δ and the β peptide chain, so that the overall resemblance between the two peptide chains is very high indeed and the differences between them explicable on the basis of the series of single mutational events, each producing a single amino acid alteration.

VARIANTS OF THE α CHAIN OF HEMOGLOBIN A_2

We have already mentioned that hemoglobin A is composed of α^A and β^A peptide chains, the superscripts indicating that these are peptide chains of the type corresponding to normal hemoglobin A. Hemoglobin A_2, on the other hand, has δ peptide chains instead of β. On the basis of the chemical evidence, the number of amino acid exchanges makes it desirable to give a new letter to the δ peptide chain in contrast to the peptide chains found in the abnormal human hemoglobins where the amino acid exchanges are single ones. Much more convincing, however, is the genetic situation which supports the concept of the hemoglobin A_2 molecule being composed of α^A and δ^{A_2} peptide chains.

We have already seen in hemoglobin Norfolk that there is an amino acid substitution in position 57 of the α peptide chain where a glycine residue is replaced by an aspartic acid residue. Only the heterozygote for this rare abnormality is known, but in his blood it has been possible to show a new minor component called hemoglobin $Norfolk_2$ in addition to hemoglobin A_2. In this heterozygote we have therefore two major components of hemoglobin and two minor components.

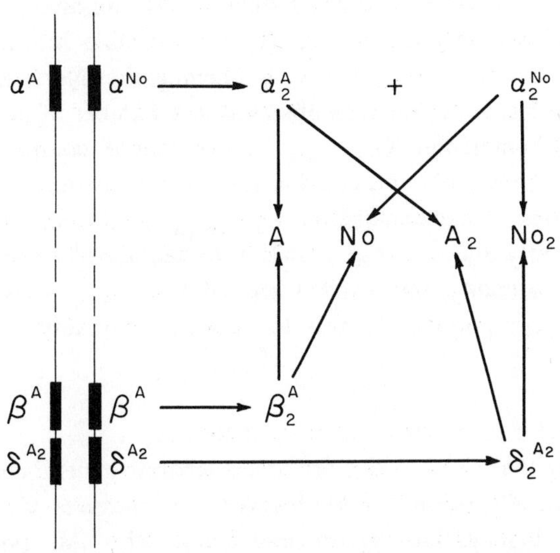

FIGURE 4-4. Genotype (left) and phenotype of the heterozygote for hemoglobin Norfolk, showing the formation of two minor components: Hb-A_2 and Hb-$Norfolk_2$
(Courtesy of Dr. C. Baglioni.)

The preliminary results (Baglioni, 1961) with fingerprinting of hemoglobin $Norfolk_2$ indicate that it has the amino acid substitution characteristic of hemoglobin Norfolk itself. In other words, the α chain of hemoglobin $Norfolk_2$ is under the same genetic control as the α chain of hemoglobin Norfolk itself. Presumably the same situation holds in a normal individual, namely that the α chains of hemoglobin A and hemoglobin A_2 are under the same genetic control. In the heterozygote for hemoglobin Norfolk the two minor components together amount to approximately 2.5 percent of the total hemoglobin. In Figure 4-4 are shown the genotype and the corresponding phenotype for this heterozygous individual. Heterozygosity is at the α chain locus, producing two types of α chain, normal and abnormal. In the dimerized form these are then freed from the ribosomes to combine with β chain dimers of which only the normal type is available (β_2^A). Thus hemoglobin A and hemoglobin Norfolk are produced. In addition the two types of α chain dimers may combine with δ chain dimers. Again, only the normal type is available resulting in two minor components hemoglobin A_2 and hemoglobin $Norfolk_2$.

The same situation has been observed in a number of instances, for example in hemoglobin $G_{Philadelphia}$ a new minor component corresponding to hemoglobin G_2 could be seen in an individual heterozygous for hemoglobin A and hemoglobin $G_{Philadelphia}$ (Stretton, unpublished). Again, recently Shooter *et al.* (1960) have had another instance of an α chain abnormality, the socalled hemoglobin G_{Ibadan} in which also a new minor component, G_2, was to be seen. Probably, this may be written as $\alpha_2^G\delta_2^{A_2}$.

VARIANTS OF THE δ CHAIN OF HEMOGLOBIN A_2

It is clear that the δ chains are under separate genetic control from the β chains. Ceppellini (1959) observed some mutants of hemoglobin A_2—called hemoglobin B_2—in individuals who did not show a simultaneous β chain abnormality. This so-called hemoglobin B_2 was found by Ceppellini to be linked genetically to the β chain locus, because in one of his families individuals occurred who were heterozygous at the δ locus for hemoglobin B_2 and at the β locus for hemoglobin S.

In Figure 4-5 the genotype and the phenotype of Ceppellini's doubly heterozygous person are shown. The α chains in this individual are normal and only one type is made, but it can be clearly seen how the two major hemoglobins A and S and the two minor hemoglobins A_2 and B_2 are formed. In this family the β chain abnormality and the δ chain abnormality although linked are in repulsion. The linkage is supported by Ceppellini's finding that the marriage of the double heterozygote in Figure 4-5 with a normal woman gave rise to six children who were either Hb S or Hb B_2 carriers. In a family of

Huisman's (1961) an abnormality of hemoglobin A_2 called hemoglobin A_2', was found to be linked to a β chain thalassemia, but this time the two mutations were in coupling. In either case, where two types of the minor component are produced together, it has been found that together they amounted to the expected figure. It looks as if each of the two δ chain loci is responsible for making a certain amount of δ chain. Although the amount of protein to be made is fixed, the

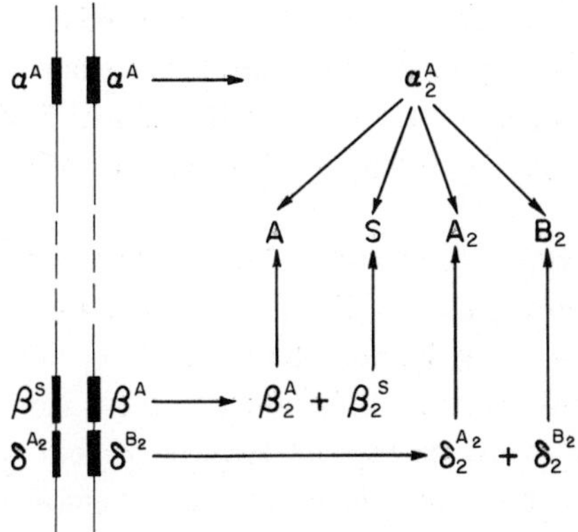

FIGURE 4-5. Genotype (left) and phenotype of Ceppellini's (1959) double heterozygote for the Hb-S and Hb-B_2 abnormalities

structure of that protein may be affected by a genetic alteration. For example, hemoglobin Norfolk does not account for 50 percent of the major hemoglobin components, but only for some 35 percent, and the same is true for some of the other abnormal hemoglobins. We have therefore to postulate altogether four structural loci in the hemoglobin system, α, β, γ, and δ. The β and δ loci seem to be closely linked, although the genetic evidence is still meager. The α locus is certainly a long way away, since it segregates independently of the β locus. We do not know, however, whether a long way away means that it could still be on the same chromosome or whether it would have to be on a different chromosome. Since no genetic abnormalities of the γ chain are known, we have no means of locating the γ chain locus in relation to the β or δ chain locus. Motulsky (1962) and Neel (1961) have suggested that γ is part of a cluster with β and δ.

GENETIC CONTROL OF HEMOGLOBIN A_2

In considering the genetic control of the production of the hemoglobin peptide chains, we note that there are four loci involved, the α, β, γ, and δ structural genes. Some of these loci are active some of the time, for example α, β, and δ are active in the adult; α and γ are active in the fetus. There must be a mechanism for turning these structural genes on and off. Whereas the α chain structural gene is active all the time; γ is turned off in the adult; β and δ are inactive in the fetus. Models for such switch mechanisms will be discussed in the next chapter.

The problem which concerns us here is the quantitative control of hemoglobin A_2 production. The following curious situation exists: the indications are that hemoglobin A and A_2 are produced in the same cell; the two proteins differ only in their β or δ peptide chains and these are distinguished by very few amino acid alterations. However, there is nearly *forty times* as much hemoglobin A made as hemoglobin A_2, without any obviously sufficient distinction between the proteins to allow one to think of feed-back controls. In looking for other types of control mechanism, we can attempt to discuss the situation in terms of the concept of an operator locus proposed by Jacob and Monod (1961) for the bacterial systems, with the reservation that the concepts may not necessarily be appropriate for our mammalian system. In Figure 4-6 are illustrated the four structural genes as straight lines, showing the length of the genetic material. In front of each is drawn the operator as a box of unknown constitution, which may be either turned off, as indicated by a cross, or which may be turned on, as indicated by the absence of a cross and the presence of an arrow. In this Figure it may be noticed that the δ chain locus does not have an operator of its own, but rather that we are postulating that the same operator controls the activity of β and δ structural genes together (see also Neel, 1961; Motulsky, 1962). This hypothetical postulate is based on the fact that in the development of the fetus there

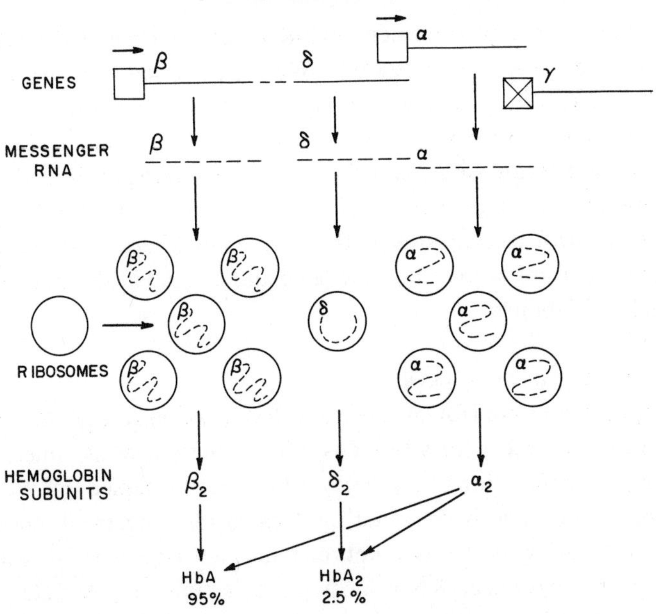

FIGURE 4-6. Scheme for control at the gene level of the quantitative difference between the rates of synthesis of hemoglobins A and A_2

is a gradual, but simultaneous, turning on of β and δ chain production, while at the same time the γ chain production declines. This is at least a suggestion of joint control of these two peptide chains. The findings in the so-called "high fetal" gene homozygote (see next chapter) also support this suggestion. In conformity with current concepts of the control of protein synthesis we may picture in Figure 4-6 that each active structural gene produces its characteristic messenger or template RNA molecule which then in turn goes to occupy a ribosome in the cytoplasm surrounding the nucleus. It is necessary to postulate that the messenger RNA leaves the nucleus, the presumed site of its synthesis and goes into the ribosomes, since it is possible to prepare cellfree systems containing only ribosomes and no nuclei which are capable of synthesizing protein. In addition we note that in the mammalian reticulocyte which is still capable of synthesizing hemoglobin and which still contains ribosomes, there is no obvious nucleus left.

The "silent" γ structural gene in the adult does not make γ chain messenger, because it is turned off. We are picturing here the control of the production of hemoglobin A_2, as a problem in the control of the production of δ peptide chains compared to β chains. In other words we are trying to explain the very great discrepancy in the rate of production of β and δ peptide chains. In terms of Figure 4-6, we can think of control mechanisms at three different levels; control at the gene level, control at the ribosome level and control at the stage of the assembly of subunits.

CONTROL AT THE GENE LEVEL

In considering control at the gene level, we may say that the β structural gene makes forty times as much β messenger as δ messenger and that therefore for every forty ribosomes occupied by β chain messengers only one is occupied by δ chain messengers. Inherent in this consideration is the assumption that each ribosome is occupied by only one messenger RNA molecule at a time, a postulate which has already been examined earlier and which we believe to be correct for the hemoglobin synthesizing system. The further assumption is also included that ribosomes have equal affinity for β and δ messenger RNA molecules. In our present state of ignorance on the relationship between ribosomes and messenger RNA we cannot judge the validity of the last assumption. This kind of control mechanism certainly presents a simple picture, since all control is located at the level of the gene and since all the rest of the scheme follows automatically. We would need a supply, a limited supply, of empty ribosomes ready to be occupied by messenger RNA molecules. We can further assume that the synthesis of the actual peptide chains themselves proceeds at the same rate for both β and δ chains, which makes sense when one considers that there is so little structural difference between these two types of peptide chain. The messenger in this scheme would be a stable messenger, capable of synthesizing a number, perhaps even a large number, of peptide chains. There is now a certain amount of evidence to indicate that the messenger RNA molecules in mammalian reticulocytes are indeed stable (Marks *et al.*, 1962). In summary, the situation that forty times as much β chain as δ chain is made is due to the fact in this scheme that the β chain genes make forty times as much messenger RNA.

However, this may be a situation peculiar to the human reticulocyte. In some animals, for example in the horse and in the mouse, there are two types of adult hemoglobin perhaps also under separate genetic control. However, the components do not seem to differ much in the quantities produced. In these cases we have no precise information yet about the chemical differences between the types of hemoglobin.

There is a difficulty in the scheme for control at the genetic level, since after all in the developing red cell there are structural genes active in the production of a variety of proteins, both structural proteins and enzyme proteins. All of the enzymes, at least, are also made in small amount. In quantitative terms the production of δ hemoglobin chains may be very similar to the production of these enzyme proteins. Perhaps we should regard the large quantities of α, β, and γ chains which can be made as extraordinarily high, rather than regarding the δ peptide chains as being abnormally slowly made. In any case, the rate at which the structural gene makes a peptide chain is in our scheme an intrinsic property of that gene which may or may not be due to some characteristic of the operator locus. However, if it turns out to be correct that β and δ chains are controlled by the same operator, then this intrinsic rate control would be more a property of the structural gene itself or the result of an interaction between the structural gene and its operator.

CONTROL AT THE RIBOSOME LEVEL

The second level of control, at the ribosome, may be considered in terms of the general scheme of peptide chain synthesis put forward by a number of people, particularly Dintzis (1961). The experimental data in his results for the synthesis of peptide chains of rabbit hemoglobin indicate a reasonably uniform growth of the chain from one end to the other. However, we know that in the δ peptide chain there are differences in amino acid structure here and there along the chain. Suppose we assume, that the presence of alanine instead of glutamic acid in position 22 causes a slowing up of peptide chain synthesis at that point. Such a control point will then be rate-controlling and although the beginning of the peptide chain could be made at a normal rate, the overall rate of synthesis and the liberation of such a peptide chain would be greatly reduced. Such a situation may be tested experimentally by performing a Dintzis type of experiment of short

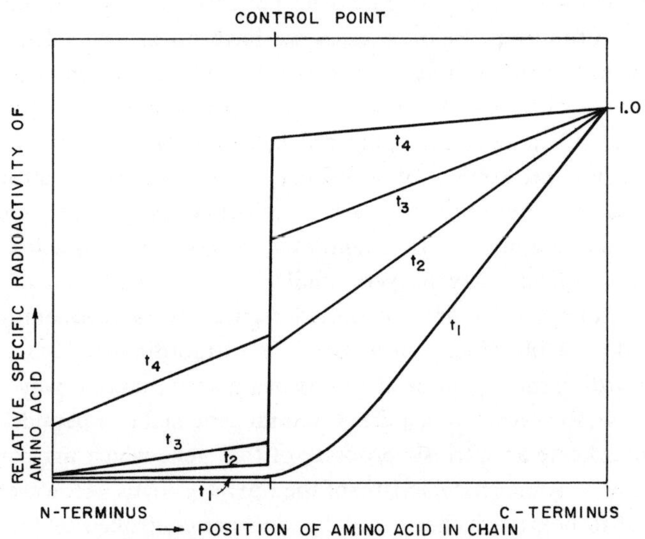

FIGURE 4-7. Diagrammatic representation of the effect of a rate controlling amino acid residue on the course of peptide chain synthesis during a pulse of a radioactive amino acid of varying duration t_1 (short), t_4 (long) The experiment is supposedly modeled after those of Dintzis (1961).

time labeling with immature human red cells. We should observe a distinct break in the plot of specific activity of amino acids against the location of such amino acids along the length of the chain (Figure 4-7).

CONTROL AT THE LEVEL OF QUARTERNARY STRUCTURE

Thirdly, we could say that there might be control of the production of δ chains at the level of the assembly of hemoglobin subunits, namely where α_2 and β_2 subunits come together to form hemoglobin A and where α_2 and δ_2 subunits come together to form hemoglobin A_2. We can postulate that the affinity of β_2 for α_2 is forty times that of δ_2 to α_2, so that on the principle of mass action far more $\alpha_2\beta_2$ is produced than $\alpha_2\delta_2$. This type of control is a function of the rate at which the subunits assemble to the final molecule; this rate would affect the rate of release of such peptide chains, or of such subunits, from their particular

$$\begin{array}{lcll} \beta \text{ RIBOSOMES} \longrightarrow & \beta_2 & & \\ & + & \rightleftharpoons & \alpha_2\beta_2 \text{ (Hb-A)} \\ \alpha \text{ RIBOSOMES} \longrightarrow & \alpha_2 & & \\ & + & \rightleftharpoons & \alpha_2\delta_2 \text{ (Hb-}A_2\text{)} \\ \delta \text{ RIBOSOMES} \longrightarrow & \delta_2 & & \end{array}$$

FIGURE 4-8. Scheme for control at the level of subunit assembly of the quantitative difference between the rate of synthesis of hemoglobins A and A_2

ribosomes (Figure 4-8). Such a scheme is a distinct possibility that also poses some difficulties of its own, particularly in certain types of thalassemia and in the so-called high fetal gene syndrome, which will be discussed in a later chapter.

HEMOGLOBIN LEPORE

This abnormal hemoglobin ($\text{Lepore}_{\text{Boston}}$) was first described by Gerald and Diamond (1958). It is slow moving and usually comprises 10 – 15 percent of total hemoglobin in the heterozygote. Heterozygosity for Lepore and for a β chain thalassemia produces a severe anemia. Other instances have been described by Neeb *et al.* (1961) $(\text{Lepore})_{\text{Hollandia}}$ and by Fessas *et al.* (1961) who call this hemoglobin Pylos. In the heterozygotes the amount of hemoglobin A_2 is reduced to about half the normal value. Homozygotes who show the symptoms of thalassemia major have been reported as having no hemoglobin A_2 at all (Fessas *et al.*, 1961). The possibility exists that hemoglobin Lepore is a δ chain mutant with its quantitative control altered so that a relatively large amount is made. Hemoglobin $\text{Lepore}_{\text{Boston}}$ and hemoglobin Pylos have been fingerprinted (Gerald *et al.*, 1961; Fessas *et al.*, 1961);

and they give patterns which are indistinguishable from those of hemoglobin A_2. That is to say, the fingerprints together with amino acid analysis (Gerald *et al.*, 1961) indicate that peptides 12, 26, and 25 have δ chain characteristics. Baglioni (1962) finds that the peptides derived from the C-terminal section of the β chain of hemoglobin $Lepore_{Boston}$ are true β chain peptides and do not carry any of the δ chain substitutions usually found there (Ingram and Stretton, 1962 and unpublished). Barnabas and Muller (1962) report for their hemoglobin Lepore ($Lepore_{Hollandia}$) that tryptic peptides 12 and 26 have the amino acid composition characteristic of the δ chain. They also state that peptide 25 is in composition like the β chain peptide.

Since the order of tryptic peptides in the human β or δ chain is $4 \cdot 12 \cdot 26 \cdot 25 \cdot \ldots$, it follows that the $Lepore_{Hollandia}$ chain has the constitution $\delta 4 \cdot \delta 12 \cdot \delta 26 \cdot \beta 25 \cdot \beta \cdot \beta \cdot$ etc. Baglioni postulates that the hemoglobin Lepore gene arose as the result of nonhomologous crossing over within the β and δ structural genes, having the information for the δ chain at the beginning and for the β chain at the end. Thus a peptide chain is made which is part δ and part β. The quantitative control mechanism, however, would be more or less that of the β chain and that is why such an unusually large amount—for a δ chain component—is made. If substantiated, this would be a most interesting example of the chemical effect of nonhomologous crossing over in the hemoglobin genetic system with far reaching consequences for our ideas on the location of the quantitative control mechanism for protein synthesis. It would be obviously reminiscent of Smithies' findings in the haptoglobins.

5

THE SWITCH FROM FETAL TO ADULT PROTEIN

It is a curious fact that the human fetus has a hemoglobin (F) which in certain quite fundamental respects is different from the adult hemoglobin (reviewed in White and Beaven, 1959). On the other hand the overall plan of the fetal hemoglobin molecule is similar to the adult hemoglobin, since it is also composed of four peptide chains (Schroeder and Matsuda, 1958; Hunt, 1959) of two different types ($\alpha_2\gamma_2$ may be written as its formula) and since each molecule of molecular weight 68,000 carries four heme groups just like adult hemoglobin. Nevertheless the differences are striking, particularly in the possession of γ instead of β peptide chains and the consequent alkali stability of fetal hemoglobin. It is not really clear why the human fetus needs a different hemoglobin. The oxygen affinity of hemoglobin F *in the fetal circulation* is higher than the oxygen affinity of the adult hemoglobin in the adult circulation. We might imagine a definite physiological advantage, because in such a system oxygen will be taken across the placental barrier from the maternal circulation into the fetus. However, it appears that this is not an intrinsic property of fetal hemoglobin, because Allen and Jandl (1960) have shown that samples of human fetal and human adult hemoglobin solutions dialyzed simultaneously against the same buffer solution result in hemoglobin solutions with the same oxygen affinity. In other words, it seems to be the interaction between fetal hemoglobin and its environment which produces the overall higher affinity of fetal blood for oxygen. It is moreover not just the hemoglobin which is different in the human fetus, but there are a number of enzymes which have different forms in the fetal and in the adult. Among other animals also there are several examples where one can easily identify the fetal hemoglobin as being chemically different from the adult hemoglobin. This is so, for example, with the monkey, ox, goat, sheep, and mouse. Possibly this list will be extended; and equally possibly those animals where a distinct difference between the fetal and adult hemoglobin has not yet been shown may in fact have such a difference which is waiting to be characterized.

In considering the change from the fetal protein to the adult protein we are considering a problem in differentiation, since we are changing a typical body protein during the embryonic development of an organism. This is indeed differentiation at the molecular level. The problem of the switch from fetal to adult hemoglobin could also be important from the point of view of certain hereditary hemoglobinopathies, such as thalassemia. In thalassemia major the affected adult may produce very considerable quantities of the fetal protein, a curious situation which we will attempt to explain later.

We have already characterized human fetal hemoglobin as $\alpha_2^A\gamma_2^F$, indicating that it contains the same two α peptide chains of the adult hemoglobin, but two rather different γ peptide chains to make up the rest of the molecule. It may well be that Perutz's model of the configuration of the hemoglobin peptide chains applies also in broad principles to fetal hemoglobin. The differences are to be sought in the amino acid sequences of the γ peptide chain which distinguish it from the β peptide chain. The most striking difference of the whole molecule, which has been known for over a hundred years, lies in the resistance of fetal hemoglobin to denaturation by acid or alkali (reviewed in White and Beaven, 1959). Hemoglobin A above pH 12 quickly undergoes irreversible changes such as the formation of a hemochromogen spectrum and insolubility when the pH is returned to neutrality. On this basis one can distinguish easily adult from fetal hemoglobin, because the fetal pigment is denatured slowly under these circumstances. Fetal hemoglobin resists the attack of alkali for a fairly long time, before anything striking happens. There are two aspects of this reaction which have been useful from a practical point of view. One is able to estimate the quantity of fetal hemoglobin in a blood sample quite easily, because after exposure to alkali for a short period of time the denatured adult hemoglobin may be easily precipitated, thus leaving the fetal protein in solution to be estimated spectrophotometrically. It is a fact, however, that the resistance of fetal hemoglobin is a resistance of the whole molecule, both α and γ peptide chains, whereas the sensitivity of hemoglobin A to the same reaction is also a property of both peptide chains, the α and β peptide chains. Thus it seems that the complexing with γ peptide chains which themselves are only moderately resistant to alkali denaturation confers the property of resistance to the α peptide chains, although these are easily attacked by the reagent when combined with β chains. Hemoglobin Barts ($= \gamma_4^F$) has only about 70 percent of the resistance of Hb F to alkali. It is the oxyhemoglobin form, that is to say hemoglobin combined with oxygen, which shows this behavior towards alkali denaturation. However, hemoglobin is also capable of combining reversably with carbonmonoxide. The carbonmonoxy hemoglobin is a very stable derivative of hemoglobin, since the protein has a very high affinity for carbonmonoxide. Carbonmonoxy adult hemoglobin is however relatively resistant to alkali denaturation. The differentiation between adult and fetal hemoglobin cannot therefore be made when the hemoglobin is in the carbonmonoxy form.

Fetal hemoglobin may also be distinguished quite easily from the adult type by electrophoresis, particularly at pH 6 in agar gel, where the fetal hemoglobin moves ahead of adult hemoglobin as a nice compact spot. Adult hemoglobin, hemoglobin A, on the other hand, seems to be adsorbed somewhat to the gel, since it forms bullet shaped spots in this type of electrophoresis. This is also true for the abnormal adult human hemoglobins.

On the basis of acid resistance of fetal hemoglobin, Betke (see Kleihauer *et al.*, 1957) developed an ingenuous method for determining whether individual red blood cells contained fetal or adult hemoglobin.

Betke prepared a smear of these red blood cells from, for example, cord blood of a newborn infant which contains a mixture of the two types of hemoglobin. The hemoglobin A inside the cells is eluted by means of a somewhat acid buffer solution which denatures the adult hemoglobin so that it becomes dissociated into lower molecular weight subunits (34,000) and is therefore able to diffuse through the cell walls to be washed away. However, the fetal hemoglobin is not

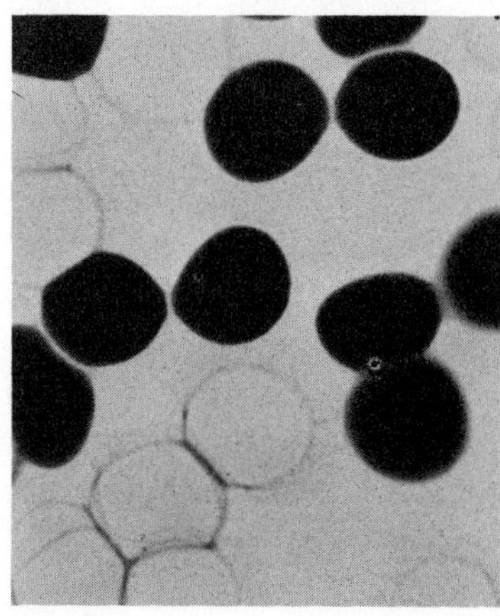

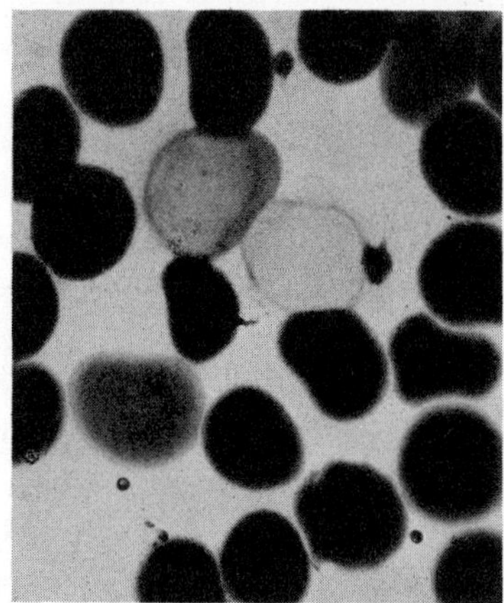

FIGURE 5-1. Estimating hemoglobins A and F in individual cells
Left: artificial mixture of cells containing either all Hb-A (ghosts) or all Hb-F (black). Right: cord blood specimen showing empty cells (Hb-A), full cells (Hb-F) and cells of intermediate staining properties which originally contained a mixture of Hb-A and Hb-F. (Kleihauer, Braun, Betke, 1957; photograph courtesy of Dr. Betke.)

affected and is retained inside the cells. If the preparation is then stained for protein, cells containing only fetal hemoglobin will stain very dark, cells containing only the adult hemoglobin will be colorless and appear as ghosts, whereas cells containing a mixture of the two proteins will be intermediate in staining color. In Figure 5-1 are shown two such stained preparations of Betke's. On the left is shown an artificial mixture of cells some containing a very high percentage of fetal hemoglobin and others containing only hemoglobin A. It may be seen that after the treatment the adult cells are empty, whereas the fetal cells are full. On the right is shown a cord blood specimen containing a mixture of the two types of hemoglobin. It will be seen that there are both empty and full cells, as well as cells containing intermediate amounts of hemoglobin. It seems that in this sample at least there is a mixed population of cells containing a range of proportions of fetal hemoglobin. The important point to note is that there are cells which appear to contain, or to have contained a mixture of both fetal and adult hemoglobin in one cell. The cell is therefore capable of producing both types of hemoglobin simultaneously and we might deduce that the switch from fetal to adult hemoglobin production is a switch of a mechanism inside the cell and not necessarily a change in the type of cell population. Itano (1957) states that in blood samples containing only hemoglobins S and F all cells can be made to sickle. This indicates that both the adult (Hb S) and the fetal hemoglobin are present together in the same cell.

Figure 5-2 is another illustration of Betke's where a cord blood specimen containing both types of hemoglobin has been treated by his elution technique. This time the slide was not stained for protein, but photographed directly with light of the right wave length to be specifically absorbed by the Soret band of hemoglobin. Again we see a mixed population of cells, some empty some full and a great many which originally must have contained a mixture of fetal and adult hemoglobin.

A further chemical characterization of fetal hemoglobin was done by Hunt (1959) who fingerprinted and compared fetal hemoglobin with hemoglobin A. There were a number of distinct differences visible among the peptides and Hunt was able to show that these all resided in the so-called γ peptide chain of fetal hemoglobin. Separated α peptide chain of hemoglobin A and F gave identical fingerprints in agreement with the concept formulated earlier that the α peptide chains are common to both hemoglobins.

If we consider what has to happen in the developing fetus to obtain first red cells with only fetal hemoglobin in them and then later on red cells with adult hemoglobin, it seems likely that there must be a switch somewhere in the life of the fetus, a switch from fetal hemoglobin to adult hemoglobin. In Figure 5-3 is illustrated the gestational age when the fetus begins to show a decrease in hemoglobin F production with a corresponding increase of the hemoglobin A production. Some people would put the appearance of the adult pigment somewhat earlier than

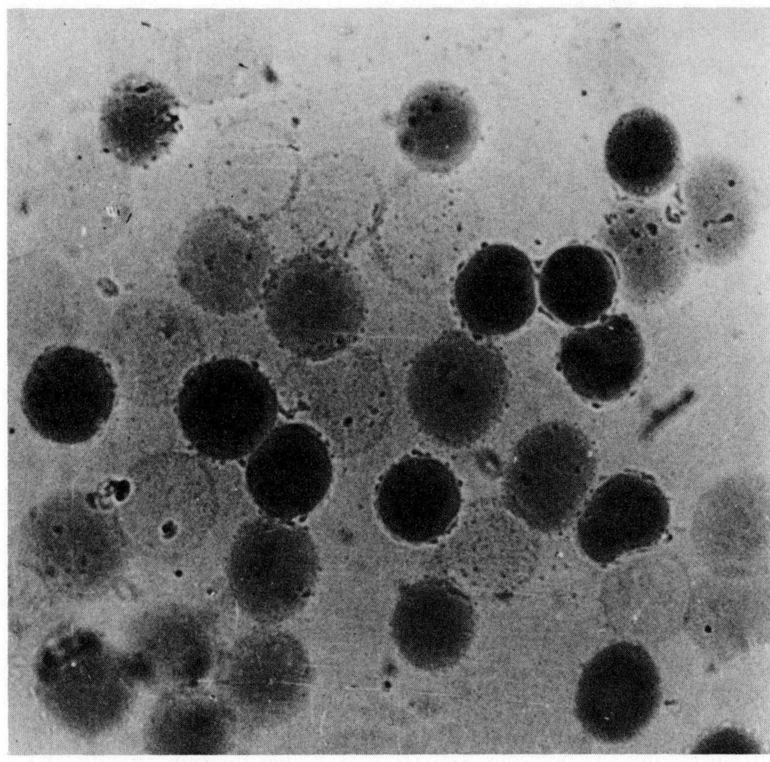

FIGURE 5-2. Estimating hemoglobins A and F in individual cells of blood as in Figure 5-1 right, but without staining

Photograph taken near the wavelength of the Soret band. (Photograph courtesy of Dr. Betke.)

thirty four weeks indicated in the figure, but then the method employed in this kind of investigation, namely alkali denaturation, is not necessarily reliable when small percentages of one or other component are involved. The precise date at which adult hemoglobin first makes its appearance must therefore remain somewhat in doubt. We can see, however, that the process begins well before birth and is not notably affected by the accident of birth itself.

Thanks largely to the work of Schroeder and his colleagues (1962) we now know the amino acid sequence of the γ chain of hemoglobin F which is illustrated in Figure 5-4. The similarity with the β peptide chain is very striking and the two chains are both 146 amino acid residues long. The percentage of similar residues between the two

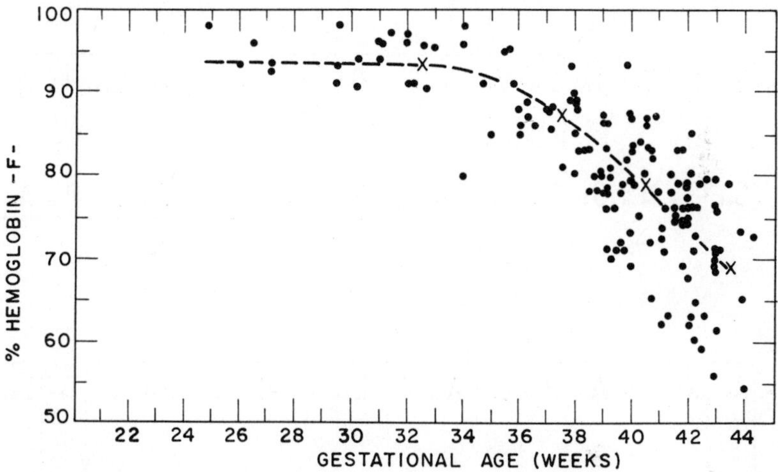

FIGURE 5-3. Percentages of fetal hemoglobin present at birth in relation to gestational age
The dotted line represents the mean percentages of fetal hemoglobin for the various gestational ages. Data represents determinations on 152 infants. (Cook *et al.*, 1957.)

chains is much greater than had been observed in the comparison of the α and β peptide chain. Altogether there are only 42 differences between β and γ as opposed to 84 between β and α. Striking, however, is the fact that alone of all the human hemoglobin peptide chains the γ chain possesses isoleucine residues, four of them. Of the regions which are similar we may notice particularly the so-called basic center (Braunitzer's term) which includes residues 59 to 66, and which is a sequence which is common to those mammalian hemoglobins which have so far been

The β and γ Peptide Chains of

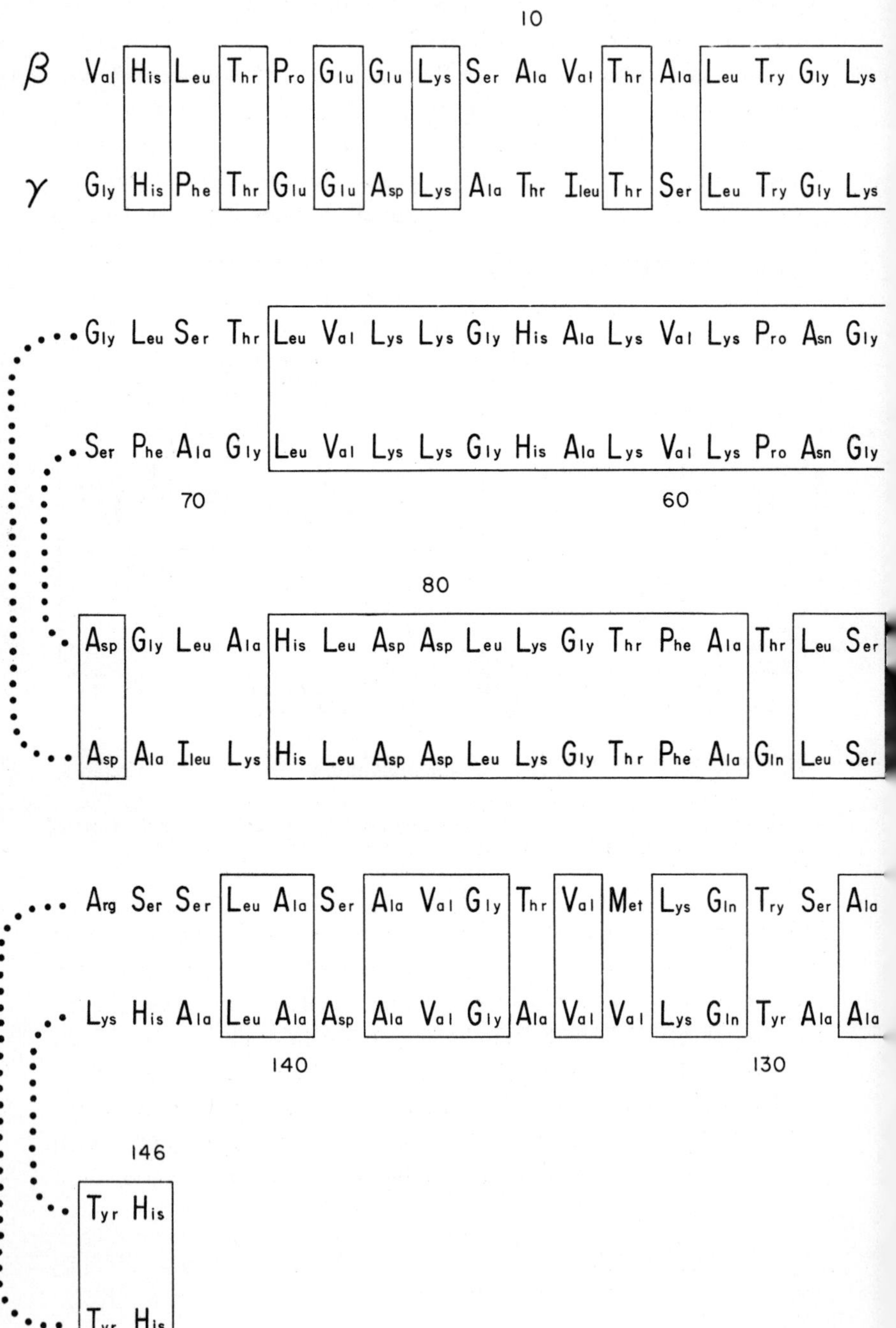

the Human Hemoglobins A and F

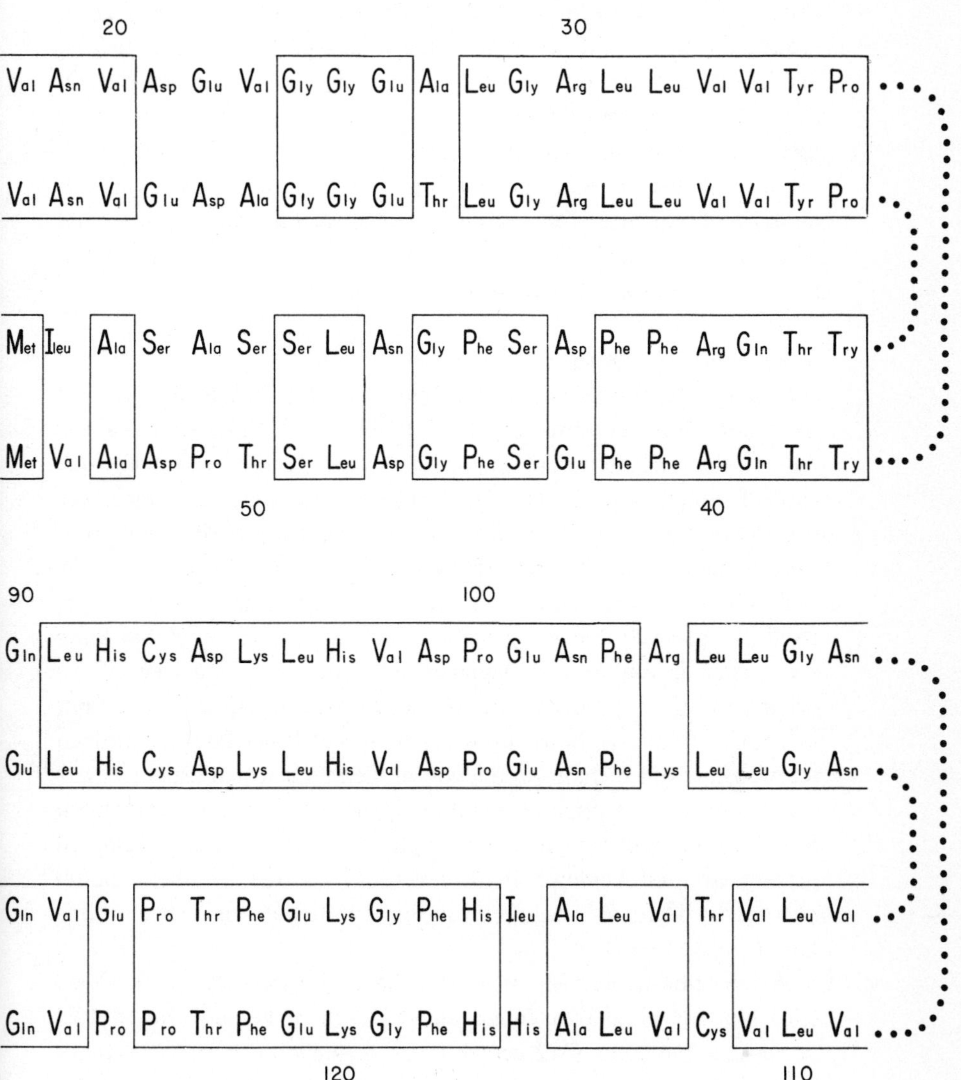

FIGURE 5-4. Sequence of amino acids in the normal human β and γ peptide chains

Identical residues are enclosed by lines. (Based on data in Figure 2-5 and Schroeder *et al.*, 1962.)

examined. On the other hand there is nothing obvious in the γ chain sequence which might account for the resistance of this chain to acid and alkali denaturation. Whether the cysteine residues in the γ chain are all present as free SH groups or whether any of them are linked by disulfide bridges is not yet quite clear. We know however that in the α and β chains there are no disulfide bonds. Even when taking the amino acid sequence of the γ chain together with the three-dimensional structure for hemoglobin and myoglobin, there is still no explanation for the extraordinary behavior of this chain.

HEMOGLOBIN F VARIANTS

In a recently published paper, Minnich *et al.* (1962) have examined by paper electrophoresis the cord blood of 90 Caucasian babies. Among them no abnormal hemoglobins were detected except for one case of hemoglobin Barts. This abnormal hemoglobin, which was first discovered by Ager and Lehmann (1958), is a protein made up of four γ peptide chains only (Hunt and Lehmann, 1959). Thus its molecular weight is normal, but its constitution is not. On the other hand it is believed that the γ chains which make up hemoglobin Barts are normal in amino acid sequence and structure. One view of the occurrence of hemoglobin Barts is that it is due to a quantitative fault in peptide chain synthesis, by which is meant genetically determined interference with α chain production in the infant which leads to overproduction of γ peptide chains and to the formation of hemoglobin Barts. The amounts of hemoglobin Barts are usually small, being 10 percent of total hemoglobin or less; as expected this hemoglobin component decreases and often vanishes by the time the infant is three months old.

In the same paper, Minnich *et al.* have also examined 449 Negro cord bloods. Here they found an incidence of hemoglobin S (10.5 percent), hemoglobin C (2 percent), and hemoglobin Barts (7 percent). These frequencies are about what is expected for an American Negro population. Again hemoglobin Barts is probably produced by an insufficiency of α chains caused possibly by the presence of the so-called α chain thalassemia. Hemoglobin A_2 in these samples was mainly between 0.1 and 1.5 percent, the normal value to be expected for a newborn infant. The precise amount of hemoglobin A_2 reported for these cord bloods is perhaps not too significant, in view of the great technical difficulties in estimating very small amounts of hemoglobin A_2. Of particular interest from our point of view is the observation that two cases of Negro cord blood (0.4 percent) showed a new abnormal fetal hemoglobin. This has been called by the authors hemoglobin $F_{\text{St. Louis}}$, because the corresponding adult hemoglobin, hemoglobin $D_{\text{St. Louis}}$, was found in one parent of each of these infants. Whilst the precise chemical abnormality which characterizes hemoglobin $D_{\text{St. Louis}}$ and hemoglobin $F_{\text{St. Louis}}$ has not yet been firmly established, there are indications from fingerprinting that in fact this abnormality is similar to, if not identical with, hemoglobin $G_{\text{Philadelphia}}$, described earlier. This fact and that the abnormality is found both as an adult hemoglobin and as a fetal hemoglobin indicates that this is an abnormality of the α peptide chain and that the α chains of the fetal and adult hemoglobin are under the same genetic control. The argument is reinforced by the fact that in the parent of each of the two babies there is both hemoglobin $D_{\text{St. Louis}}$ and also a so-called split A_2 minor component. This indicates, as it did in hemoglobin Norfolk, that since the parent is heterozygous for hemoglobin A and hemoglobin $D_{\text{St. Louis}}$, at the α locus, in him two A_2 components are produced, hemoglobin A_2 and hemoglobin D_2. Again this is consistent with the formulation of an α chain abnormality and that the α chains of hemoglobin A, A_2, and F are all controlled by the same gene (see also Baglioni *et al.*, 1961).

In Figure 5-5 we see at the top the development of various types of hemoglobin in patient DW (taken from the paper of Minnich *et al.*) in the course of the first twelve months of this infant's life. The genotype of this particular infant may be written as:

$$\frac{\alpha^{A}}{\alpha^{A}}\,\frac{\beta^{S}}{\beta^{A}}\,\frac{\gamma^{F}}{\gamma^{F}}\,\frac{\delta^{A_2}}{\delta^{A_2}}$$

At first the blood contains over 80 percent of fetal hemoglobin which drops to a few percent at twelve months. At the same time the production of the two adult hemoglobins, hemoglobin A and S, rises

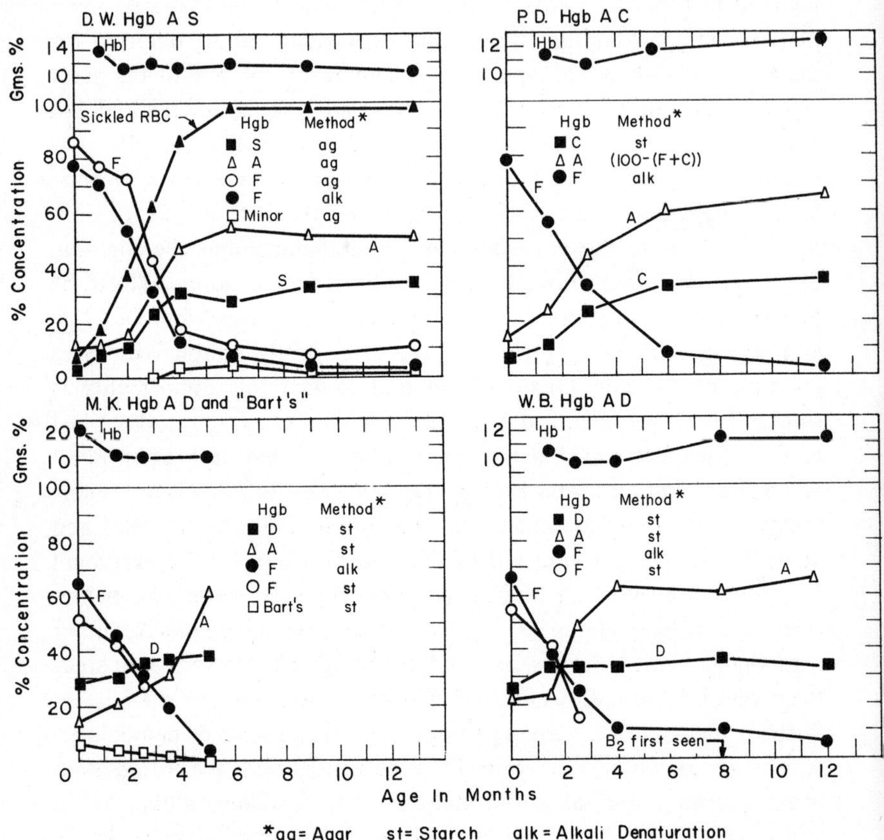

FIGURE 5-5. Changes with age in the concentration of hemoglobins of infants with hemoglobins S, C, and $D_{St. Louis}$
"The minor component shown for D.W. is the one described by Robinson *et al.* (1957) with a mobility between that of Hb-A and Hb-F. Hemoglobin B_2 in W.B. is the abnormal component described by Ceppellini (1959)." By permission from V. Minnich *et al.*, *Blood* 19: 137 (1962), published by Grune and Stratton, New York.

simultaneously and in parallel. Both the genes involved, β^{A} and β^{S}, have been switched on apparently at the same time. There is also a rise of the percentage of sickled cells in the sickling test which increases from almost 0 at birth to sickling of all the cells by the time the infant is six months old. This is, of course, due to the presence in this blood sample of hemoglobin S in these cells. The fact that practically all the cells can be made to sickle in this test indicates that all cells contain both hemoglobin A and hemoglobin S side by side.

Patient MK in Figure 5-5 on the other hand is the result of a different genotype, namely:

$$\frac{\alpha^{D}}{\alpha^{A}}\ \frac{\beta^{A}}{\beta^{A}}\ \frac{\gamma^{F}}{\gamma^{F}}\ \frac{\delta^{A_2}}{\delta^{A_2}}$$

This time there is heterozygosity at the α chain locus. We can see that at birth this infant had 60 percent of fetal hemoglobin, which dropped to almost zero by six months. As before, the hemoglobin A component, determined by quantitative electrophoresis, rises from a low value to about 60 percent. The rise of hemoglobin A parallels the fall of hemoglobin F. Also present is hemoglobin D determined by electrophoresis. This, however, remains almost constant rising only slightly after birth, yet at the same time the fetal hemoglobin component determined by alkali denaturation falls. The explanation given by the authors is that at birth the electrophoretic D component is really hemoglobin $F_{St.\ Louis}$ which may be written as $\alpha_2^{D}\gamma_2^{F}$. This is then replaced by the adult counterpart, hemoglobin $D_{St.\ Louis}$ which may be written as $\alpha_2^{D}\beta_2^{A}$. The method of electrophoresis used by the authors cannot distinguish between hemoglobin $F_{St.\ Louis}$ and hemoglobin $D_{St.\ Louis}$ and they are therefore recorded as one component.

The fingerprinting examination which was carried out was done unfortunately only on the adult hemoglobin $D_{St.\ Louis}$ and it is this component which shows the chemical similarity with the α chain mutant hemoglobin $G_{Philadelphia}$. Not enough of hemoglobin $F_{St.\ Louis}$ was available to the authors for further chemical characterization. However, their argument that such a fetal hemoglobin exists is rather convincing. In addition there may be seen a small component of hemoglobin

Barts (γ_4^F). In this case the presence of the α chain abnormality results in relatively less production of α peptide chains and overproduction of γ peptide chains. That the α chains of hemoglobin $D_{St. Louis}$ are not made as readily as α^A chains may be seen in the fact that the final percentage at twelve months is 40 percent hemoglobin D and 60 percent hemoglobin A. At about eight months a new minor hemoglobin component (B_2) was observed. This would correspond to a hemoglobin of the constitution $\alpha_2^D\delta_2^{A_2}$. It should be noted incidentally that an abnormal hemoglobin corresponding to δ_4 has now been observed (Huehns and Dance, 1962); the corresponding adult type (β_4^A) is well known as hemoglobin H. This latter seems to be produced in individuals where there is interference with α chain production such as in α chain thalassemia.

A somewhat similar abnormal fetal hemoglobin has been described by Ranney *et al.* (1962). Hemoglobin $I_{Burlington}$ in an adult could be formulated as $\alpha_2^I\beta_2^A$. The cord blood from the son of such an individual had a fetal hemoglobin fast in electrophoresis which is formulated as $\alpha_2^I\gamma_2^F$. The authors were able to show that this was a fetal hemoglobin by its alkali resistance, the presence of both valine (α) and glycine (γ) amino end groups and by the presence of isoleucine.

So far there has been no clear evidence for an abnormal fetal hemoglobin with a defect in the γ chain.

THALASSEMIA

We now turn to a discussion of the important inherited disease thalassemia. It is estimated that in Italy alone there are some two million people carrying at least one thalassemia gene (Ager and Lehmann, 1960), that is to say, they are heterozygous for thalassemia. However, the disease is certainly not confined to this area and is found in many parts of the world (see Figures 5-6 and 5-7). Thalassemia is an inherited disease in the sense that it exists in two forms: thalassemia major and thalassemia minor (see in Bianco *et al.*, 1952). Thalassemia major is a homozygous condition, whereas thalassemia minor is the corresponding heterozygous state. Whilst sickle-cell anemia seems to be a fairly well defined single entity, thalassemia is not; it covers a group of diseases which share certain properties, but which are expressed in different ways in different localities. For a review of the history of the

Milano (1.3)
Padova (2)
Torino (0.9)
Ferrara (7.3)
Genova (1.5)
Rovigo (9.7)
Codorigo (15.6)
Ravenna (3.7)
Bologna (0.8)
Firenze (0.4)
Ancona (1.6)
CORSICA
?
Roma (1.6)
Napoli (1.7)
Lecce (6.2)
Torre
Annunziata (2.7)
SARDINIA
Palermo (4.4)
Reggio
Calabria (3.5)
Agrigento (7.6)
Siracusa (4.2)
SICILY

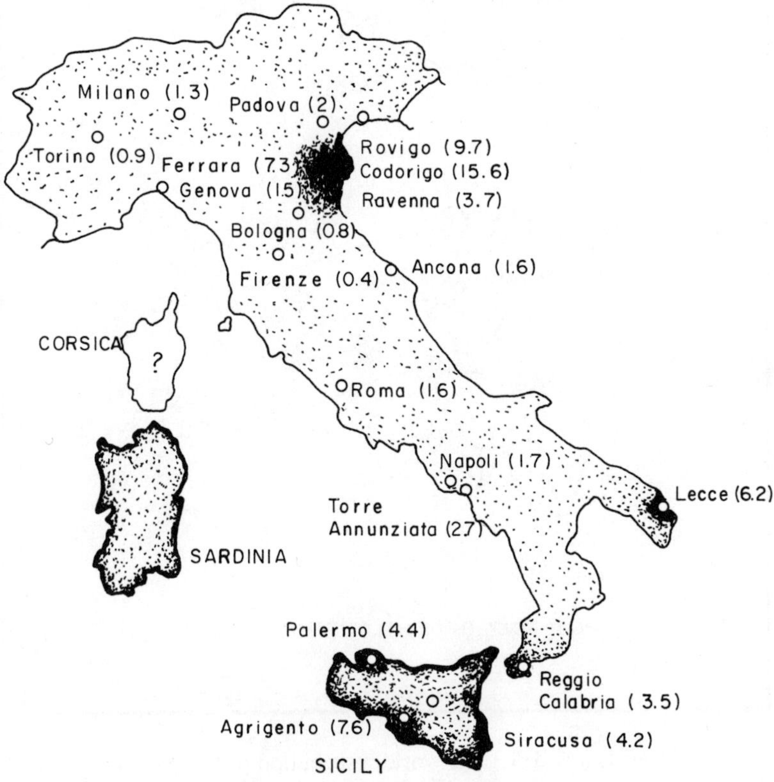

FIGURE 5-6. The distribution of thalassemia heterozygotes in Italy, from the data of Silvestroni and colleagues
The figures give the percent incidence in the various districts shown. By permission from R. M. Bannerman, *Thalassemia* (New York, Grune and Stratton, 1961).

disease and of the chemical studies on thalassemia, the reader is recommended to go to an excellent monograph recently published by Bannerman (1962).

Thalassemia major was first clearly described by Cooley in 1925 and is in fact often called Cooley's anemia. The name thalassemia derived

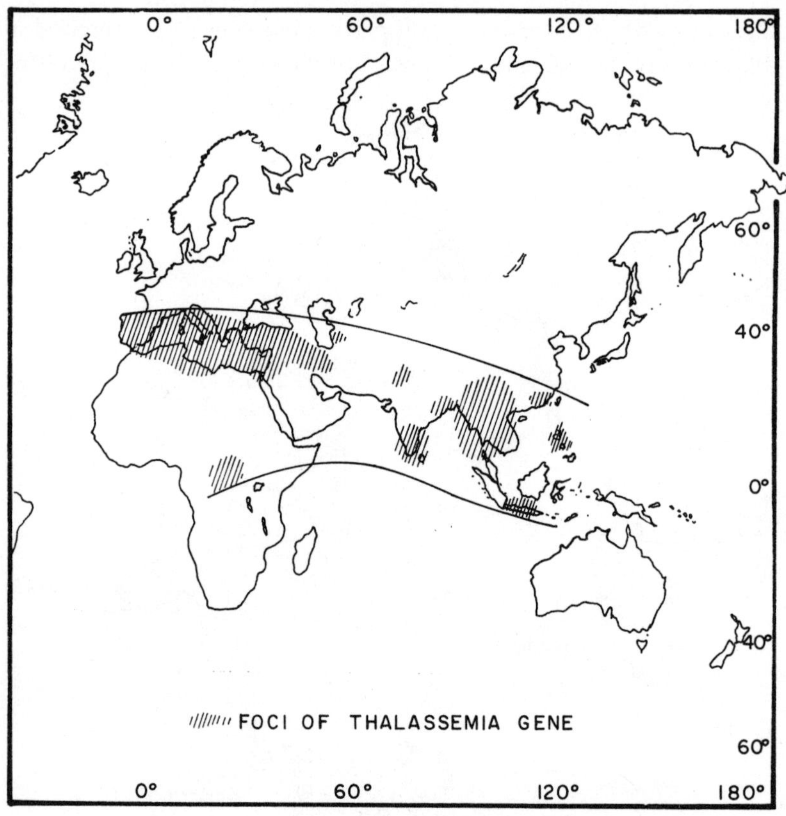

FIGURE 5-7. The world distribution of thalassemia
By permission from A. I. Chernoff, *Blood* 14: 899 (1959), published by Grune and Stratton, New York.

from the fact that it is found in high frequency in the Mediterranean area (*thalassos*, the sea). It is considered by many people that the major factor in thalassemia is a deficiency in hemoglobin production within the cells. As a result the cells may be too small or too thin and are readily eliminated from the circulation. Somehow the spleen recognizes such cells as being abnormal and destroys them, although this may not be the only way in which these cells are lost. A severe hemolytic anemia results.

As in sickle-cell anemia, homozygous thalassemia is a very serious condition and most of the people possessing it do not live to reproductive age in their native habitat. Again malaria is called in to explain the extraordinarily high frequency of such a seriously deleterious gene. Again it is postulated that somehow the heterozygote possesses some selective advantage with respect to malaria which would lead to an increase in the number of thalassemia genes in the population. This cannot be the complete explanation, however, because there are a number of areas in Italy for example which have been in the past highly malarious and which do not contain appreciable numbers of thalassemia (Bannerman, 1962). Since we must assume that there are several genetic forms of thalassemia, we must also assume that they have arisen independently in a number of localities. We will see later that we can classify thalassemia into α and β chain thalassemias, but then in each of these two groups there is probably a diversity of forms having arisen from a number of independent mutational events.

Various theories have been advanced to explain the molecular mechanism of thalassemia. One theory elaborated in Bannerman (1962) proposes that the genetic block occurs somewhere along the line of synthesis of the heme group. It is postulated that either there is interference during the synthesis of the protoporphyrin ring or possibly interference at the last stage of synthesis which involves putting an iron atom in the center of the heme group. In any case, on the basis of this hypothesis, there is insufficient heme available and therefore there is a reduction in the total amount of hemoglobin made per cell. This would be so in spite of the fact that iron itself is readily available and indeed would be expected to accumulate, as it does in a typical thalassemia major. It will be seen later, however, that other explanations can be produced for this phenomenon. Whilst it is possible that some instances of thalassemia are caused by such an interference with heme synthesis, this is not likely to be the case for that kind of thalassemia (interacting thalassemia) found together with some abnormal hemoglobins. It is also not clear why there is not also an accumulation of peptide chains or of globin in the cells as there should be on the basis of Bannerman's hypothesis. We would have to assume further that there is independent control for the rate of synthesis of globin and of heme.

THALASSEMIA: A STRUCTURAL MUTATION

Another theory originally proposed by Itano (1957) and more recently elaborated by Ingram and Stretton (1959) postulates a genetic interference with the production of the protein peptide chains. We would postulate that just as an abnormal hemoglobin is made at a slower rate, so in thalassemia there might be an amino acid substitution or other structural alteration which reduces the rate of production of the hemoglobin protein. Since, however, the hemoglobin in thalassemia is known to be electrophoretically normal, we would have to postulate an amino acid substitution which does not involve an electrophoretic change. Alternatively, we would have to suppose that the abnormal hemoglobin is not made at all and therefore has not been examined. In such a view a nonelectrophoretic mutation might occur either in the α or in the β peptide chain and we would recognize two classes of thalassemia, α chain thalassemias and β chain thalassemias. In the one case, α chain production would be curtailed and such phenomena as the occurrence of hemoglobin H (Rigas *et al.*, 1955) in the adult or hemoglobin Barts (Ager and Lehmann, 1958) in the infant might be the result. Homozygous α chain thalassemias would be expected to be very rare, since they would interfere also with fetal hemoglobin and greatly endanger the life of the fetus. On the other hand, a β chain thalassemia would be expected to be more common, since it would not affect the production of fetal hemoglobin. There is therefore the possibility as originally suggested by Rich (1952) that a thalassemia major might compensate for his hemolytic anemia by producing fetal hemoglobin. Certainly hemoglobin F ($\alpha_2\gamma_2$) is found in high percentage in cases of thalassemia major which we would classify genetically as β chain thalassemias. We would also expect the proportion of hemoglobin A_2 to rise in the case of a β chain thalassemia, particularly in the heterozygote, since the δ chain production is not affected and since therefore the relative proportion of β to δ chains would be altered in favor of the δ chain. Characteristically in such thalassemias, hemoglobin A_2 is increased to a percentage of 5 – 7 percent (Kunkel *et al.*, 1957). On the other hand, in the α chain thalassemia no such rise of hemoglobin A_2 would be expected, since α chains are in short supply, and indeed none is found.

THALASSEMIA: A DEFECT IN THE CONTROL MECHANISM

There is another possibility. We might suggest that interference is not by way of a structural alteration, but is rather one involving the whole regulatory system. If there is indeed an operator control over the structural genes, then there might be a mutation in that operator gene of such a nature that any messenger or rather any ribosome containing messenger from such a gene is either incapable or not so capable of producing hemoglobin.

In the interacting β chain thalassemia, such as is found in sickle-cell thalassemia disease, it would seem unlikely that interference with heme production as postulated by Bannerman (1962) could *differentially* affect the production of hemoglobin A without also simultaneously reducing the amount of hemoglobin S made. We have to account here for the fact that sickle-cell hemoglobin is produced together with fetal hemoglobin, but that no hemoglobin A is produced. In a hemoglobin A/S heterozygote both hemoglobin A and hemoglobin S are made, but in the thalassemia heterozygote hemoglobin A production has been knocked out (see also Lehmann, 1957). The β chain thalassemia, however, does not affect the production of fetal hemoglobin.

In the so-called noninteracting type of thalassemia, where thalassemia, hemoglobin A and hemoglobin S are present side by side, a different genetic mechanism seems to be operating. The genotype in this case would be:

$$\frac{\alpha^{Th}}{\alpha^{A}}\,\frac{\beta^{A}}{\beta^{S}}\,\frac{\gamma^{F}}{\gamma^{F}}\,\frac{\delta^{A_2}}{\delta^{A_2}}$$

Here there is both a normal α and a normal β chain gene present and normal hemoglobin A is made together with hemoglobin S. This is not such a serious clinical condition and very little, if any, fetal hemoglobin is produced.

A homozygous α chain thalassemia has recently been reported from

Malaya by Lie-Enjo (1961). She found several cases of severe hydrops in newborn infants of Chinese origin who died very quickly after birth. In a number of instances it was clear that the parents carried the stigmata of thalassemia which in the Chinese population is generally considered to be an α chain thalassemia. The remarkable finding was reported that the hemoglobin contents of the infants was largely made up of hemoglobin Barts, (γ_4^F), almost entirely in fact. Presumably these infants were homozygous for an α chain type thalassemia, since the α chain production was so greatly reduced that only γ chains are made. This also implies that γ chain production is not controlled by whether or not α chains are available for combination to the final hemoglobin molecule. While the γ chain production proceeds independently in its quantitative aspects, the same may well be true of the control of β chain production, since β_4^A (hemoglobin H) is also found in α chain thalassemia. Conversely it is possible that the production of α chains is controlled by the amounts of β chains and/or γ chains available, especially since no instance of α_4 hemoglobin has so far been reported. That is to say that the release of α_2 subunits from the ribosomes depends on the presence of β_2 and γ_2 subunits.

It seems likely that most types of thalassemia are mutations which somehow or other affect the β structural genes, including perhaps a nonelectrophoretic mutation that contains amino acid substitutions not involving a change in charge. On the other hand, three such suspected samples of hemoglobin from α chain thalassemias and β chain thalassemias have been examined in great detail by Guidotti (unpublished) who has analyzed quantitatively the amino acid content of individual tryptic peptides from isolated chains. In no case could he show an amino acid alteration. However, a negative result is not necessarily conclusive. It may be that thalassemia is a deletion of the structural β chain gene or α chain gene such that the messenger RNA or the intact peptide chains cannot be made. Or again it may be a mutation in the operator locus (see Figure 4-6) which controls the α or β chain gene, such that defective β chain messenger or the α chain messenger are made. This last possibility will be explored more fully in the following section.

THE SWITCH MECHANISM FROM FETAL TO ADULT HEMOGLOBIN

We now turn to some speculations on the switch mechanism which exists in the red blood cells and which ensures that adult hemoglobin will be made in the adult and that fetal hemoglobin will be made in the fetus (Neel, 1961; Motulsky, 1962). In Figure 5-8 are illustrated in diagrammatic fashion the relative proportions of α, β, and γ peptide chains made in the red cells of a developing human fetus and newborn.

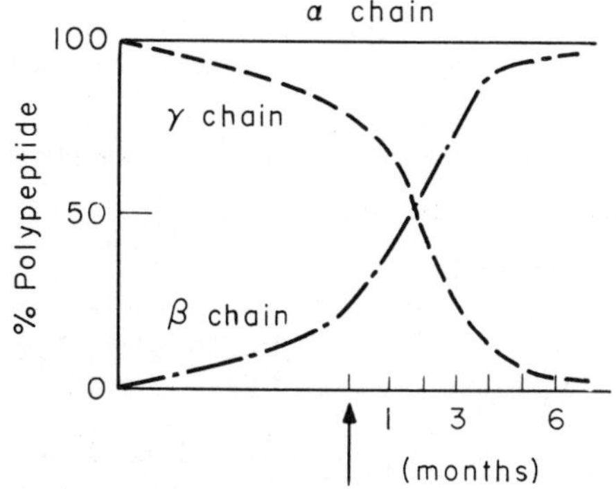

FIGURE 5-8. Diagram of the changes with age in α, β, and γ chain production in the human fetus and infant
The arrow marks the birth.

It must be remembered that the α chain is concerned in both fetal and adult hemoglobin, that the γ chain is part of the fetal hemoglobin molecule and that the β chain is characteristic of the adult protein.

In this simplified picture the production of α chain remains constant throughout the whole process. On the other hand, there is initially a manufacture of γ chains which then decreases and eventually goes down to almost zero by the time the infant has reached six months of age or so. More or less at the same time there is an increase in production of the β peptide chains of the adult hemoglobin type. This is equivalent to saying that the α chain structural gene is turned on all the time, but that the γ gene is gradually turned off, whereas the β chain gene is slowly turned on.

One way in which this phenomenon may be examined is in the light of the scheme for the control of protein synthesis which has been proposed by Jacob and Monod (1961) (Figure 5-9). This is a mechanism which ensures the activity or inactivity of structural genes within a cell.

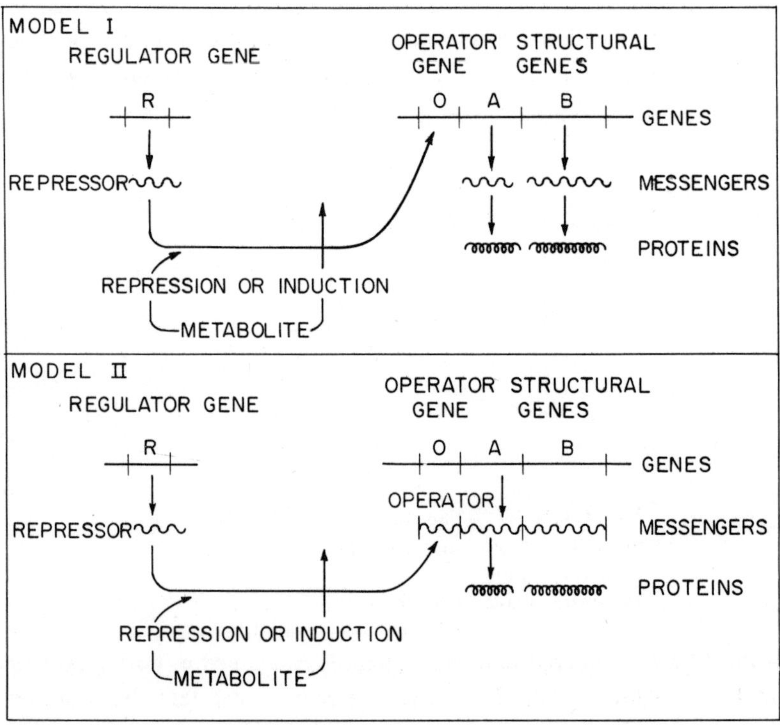

FIGURE 5-9. Models for the regulation of protein synthesis (Jacob and Monod, 1961.)

The scheme itself is derived from Jacob and Monod's studies in bacterial systems, where there is genetic evidence for more than one type of gene to be involved in the production of specific proteins. In addition to the structural gene which carries the information to produce peptide chains of specific amino acid sequences, it has become necessary to postulate the operator genes which turn structural genes on or off and also regulator genes which in turn control the activity of the operator genes.

Although we will take our model from Jacob and Monod's work, reference should be made to McClintock's (1956) earlier work in maize which led to postulated genetic elements similar to the regulator and operator genes. For our present discussion we will use the model I illustrated in Figure 5-9, rather than model II. In applying the scheme to a mammalian cell, we are of course exposing ourselves to a number

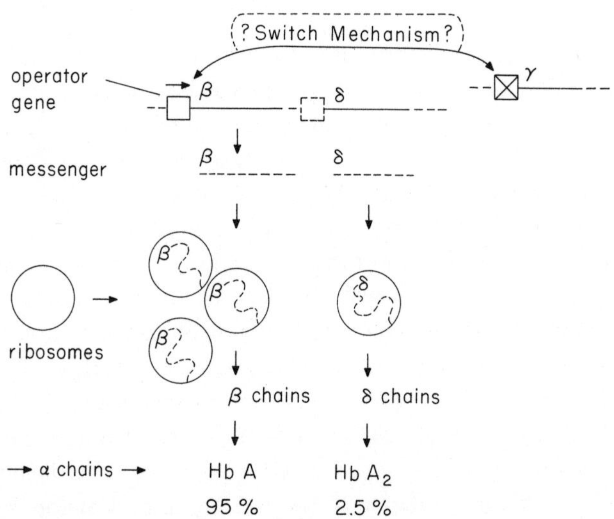

FIGURE 5-10. Model for the regulation of hemoglobin A and A_2 synthesis in the normal adult

of risks, since there is no genetic evidence at present for the presence of operator or regulator genes in the mammalian cells. A possible exception is the occurrence of the so-called "high fetal" gene to be discussed later, but even this is open to an alternative interpretation. Even if it is found eventually, that Jacob and Monod's scheme does not apply precisely to the mammalian system, it serves for the time being as a convenient and stimulating model for designing experiments.

In this scheme (Figure 5-10) each structural gene in its active state makes template molecules of the so-called "messenger RNA" type which leave the nucleus and go into the ribosomes of the cytoplasm;

there peptide chains are made on them. Whether or not these genes are active will depend on the state of their particular operator genes. The concept that several structural genes are controlled by the same operator gene, which has been developed in microorganisms may apply to two of the hemoglobin peptide chain genes, namely the β and the δ genes. On the other hand the α and β genes are controlled by independent operator genes, since these genes segregate independently.

DIFFERENTIATION AS A SWITCH MECHANISM

Baglioni (1962) has very recently proposed an explanation of the fetal–adult hemoglobin switch mechanism (Figure 5-11). Although not all the stages of maturation of red cells are agreed upon by everybody, nevertheless it seems that they spring from a pool of undifferentiated continuously dividing "stem cells" in the erythropoetic tissues of either fetus or adult. In the normal situation, a proportion of stem cells differentiate into red cell precursors (erythroblasts). These precursors may then either continue to divide or they may differentiate through a number of stages to the final mature erythrocyte. It would seem, however, that hemoglobin synthesis begins when the stem cell turns into an erythroblast. Presumably, in terms of the model which we have been using, at this stage the cell is "set" for either hemoglobin F or hemoglobin A production, or for making both. Baglioni assumes that all the hemoglobin genes are repressed in the stem cells and that they become "derepressed" or "activated" specifically (α and γ only, or α and β and δ only) as the stem cell differentiates. Whether β and δ or whether γ become derepressed, or all three, depends in this theory on the number of cell divisions previously undergone by the stem cell in question and/or on the length of time spent by the cell in that particular environment before differentiation. In the normal adult, the differentiating stem cells are sufficiently "old," so that only β and δ genes are derepressed, in addition to α genes of course. On the contrary, in the young fetus, the differentiating stem cell derepresses only the α and γ genes. At later stages of fetal life, apparently all hemoglobin genes are turned on by stem cells of intermediate "age" and for a time cells mature which contain both fetal and adult hemoglobin.

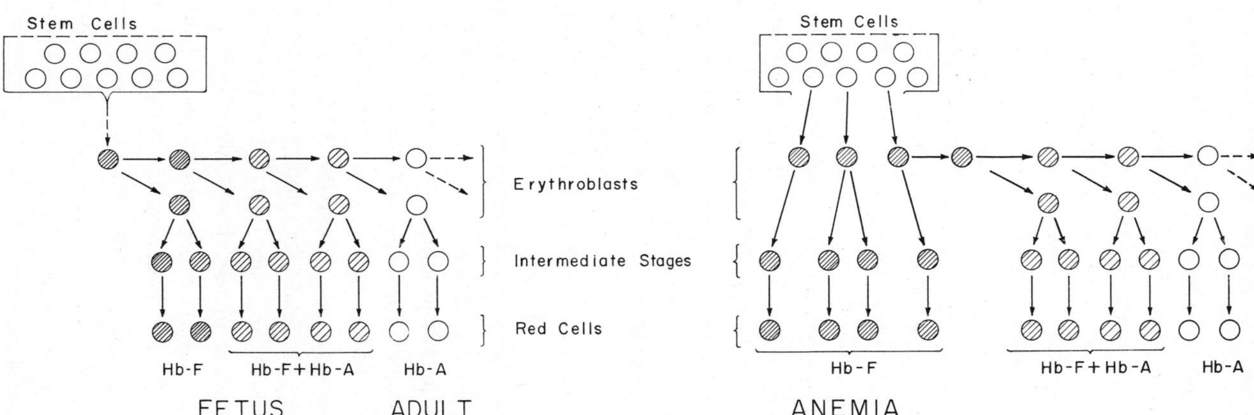

FIGURE 5-11. Model of red cell differentiation

Shown is the switch from Hb-F to Hb-A production at the end of fetal life (left) and the mechanism by which Hb-F is produced in severe anemia (right). The intensity of shading illustrates the relative amounts of Hb-F synthesized by red cell precursors at different stages of differentiation, or contained in the red cells. (Baglioni, 1962.)

There are however occasions where an adult will produce fetal hemoglobin. In the case of a severe hemolytic anemia, like sickle-cell anemia or thalassemia, the amounts of fetal hemoglobin are large and may reach almost 100 percent in thalassemia. In terms of the above theory for the switch mechanism, one would say that in a hemolytic situation large additional numbers of red cells are needed. In response, a higher proportion of stem cells mature, thus depleting the pool and causing "young" cells to differentiate; young, that is, in terms of either cell divisions undergone or time spent before differentiating. Such cells would make predominantly fetal hemoglobin. The same situation would hold true for the anemia due to excessive bleeding, although here the amounts of fetal hemoglobin are much less. There is some evidence (Latja and Oliver, 1960) that in animals made anemic by bleeding a larger number of stem cells differentiate rapidly. This is of course not enough to prove the theory, but it is certainly suggestive.

There have been suggestions (Allen and Jandl, 1960; Thomas *et al.*, 1960) that the change in oxygen tension at birth activates β chain synthesis; or that hormones may do so (Rucknagel and Chernoff, 1955). However it is difficult to explain fetal hemoglobin production in adults on the basis of such suggestions.

We might extend Baglioni's scheme in terms of the Jacob and Monod repressors and operators. We would then postulate that in the "young" stem cell of the fetus there is present a genetically controlled repressor substance capable of repressing the operator locus which controls both the β and the neighboring δ genes. These are therefore set to "silent" whilst α and γ genes become derepressed when this particular cell differentiates. Thus $\alpha_2\gamma_2$ = fetal hemoglobin is produced. However, this specific β/δ repressor is either unstable or becomes diluted out as the *stem cell* continues to divide. Eventually it is at a low level and, when *this* cell differentiates, the repressor of β and δ is inactive or absent and the β and δ loci are derepressed. In addition we must assume further that either a new repressor for the γ operator begins now to be made or that the β chain messenger RNA molecules which are produced themselves act as repressors on the γ operator. This would be a kind of feedback situation.

To account for the production of fetal hemoglobin in thalassemia, or any other hemolytic situation, we would again fall back on Baglioni's suggestion (Figure 5-11) of the forced differentiation of "young" stem cells still containing the original repressor molecules.

In an alternative scheme, we might postulate that a repressor substance for the γ operator is present all the time in these cells, but

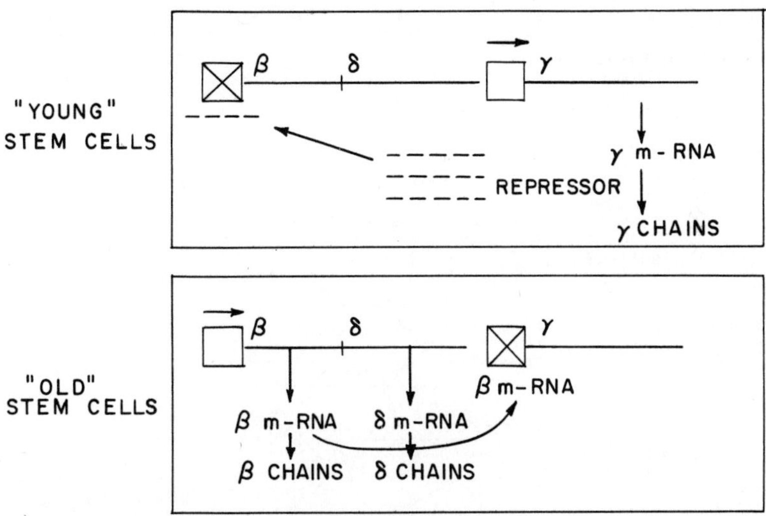

FIGURE 5-12. Model I for the mechanism which controls the switch from Hb-F to Hb-A production at the end of fetal life

that there is in addition another substance, possibly of low molecular weight, possibly some hormone, which combines with the repressor and modifies it so that the *complex* acts as a repressor for the β/δ operator, but does not act on the γ operator. During the maturation of the fetus, the stem cells gradually lose this second substance, this repressor modifier, and the repressor itself now acts to repress the γ chain operator, but is no longer active on the β operator. Such a modified scheme (Figure 5-13) would relieve the β chain messenger RNA of its dual role and might also indicate a possible involvement of hormonal substances in the switch mechanism.

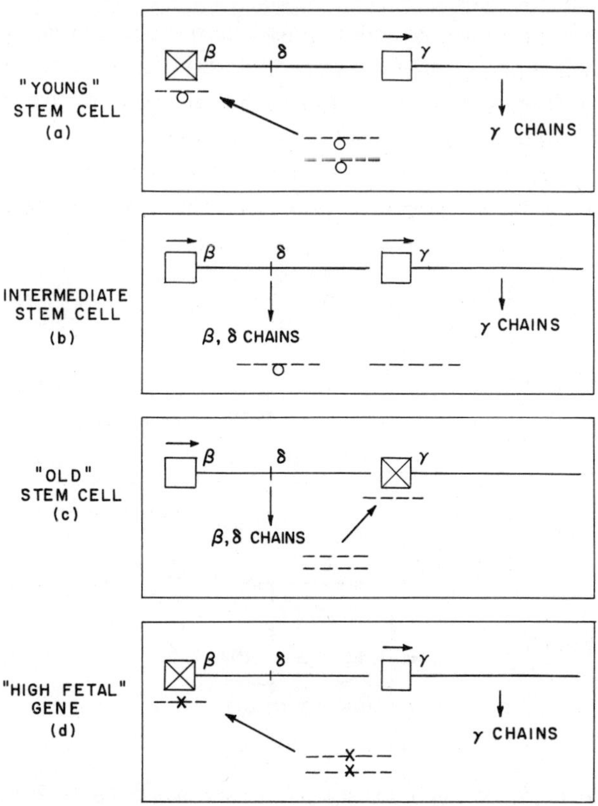

FIGURE 5-13. Model II for the mechanism which controls the switch from Hb-F to Hb-A production at the end of fetal life and in the "high fetal" gene condition
(a) Repressor type: $--\overline{0}--$
(b) Two repressor types: $--\overline{0}--$ and $-----$, neither in sufficient concentration.
(c) Repressor type: $-----$
(d) Mutated repressor: $--X--$, which can no longer combine with 0, but has now the specificity to combine with the β/δ operator, unlike $-----$.

There is some slight evidence for the influence of hormones in the production of fetal hemoglobin, since there are instances in the literature of women with false or molar pregnancies who form small amounts of fetal hemoglobin in their blood during their "pregnancy." Removal of the mole eliminates fetal hemoglobin production. It is known that during such molar pregnancies there is considerable production of a variety of hormones, particularly gonadotrophin. This is not to say, of course, that gonadotrophin itself might be involved or that indeed any hormones are necessarily involved, but it does provide another view of this important problem.

As yet another alternative, we can picture as in Figure 5-14, that the repressor modifier substance slowly increases during the change from "young" stem cells to "old" stem cells. Again the modifier could well be a low molecular weight substance arriving in the cell from the outside, although this is a more difficult concept than the gradual loss of such material from the cell (Figure 5-13). Apart from this difficulty, the scheme works equally well, with the unmodified repressor having specificity to combine with, and turn off, the β/δ operator and with the modified repressor having specificity only for the γ operator. The repressor mutation postulated for the high fetal gene in 5-13, 5-14 will be discussed later.

CONTROL MECHANISMS AND THALASSEMIA

Now we can apply these ideas on the control mechanisms to the situation in thalassemia major, where there is very considerable production of fetal hemoglobin in the adult and where there is therefore a pathological involvement of the switch mechanism. In Figure 5-15 is shown the scheme as it might apply to a homozygote suffering from a β chain thalassemia. The production of α chains is not affected. On the other hand we can assume that there is a genetic defect in the structural β chain gene such that a *defective β chain messenger* is made. There are various ways in which such a messenger might be defective; either by way of a mutation leading to an amino acid substitution not involving a change in the charge of the molecule, but preventing or at least curtailing the production of β peptide chains (Itano, 1957; Ingram and Stretton, 1959); or again the mutation in the β chain messenger might be of a more drastic type such as a deletion, with the effect that the defective β chain messenger cannot make β peptide chains. It is an essential part of this scheme that a defective β chain messenger is made and that it occupies and *blocks ribosomes*. In this way, and particularly if there are many β chain messengers made by

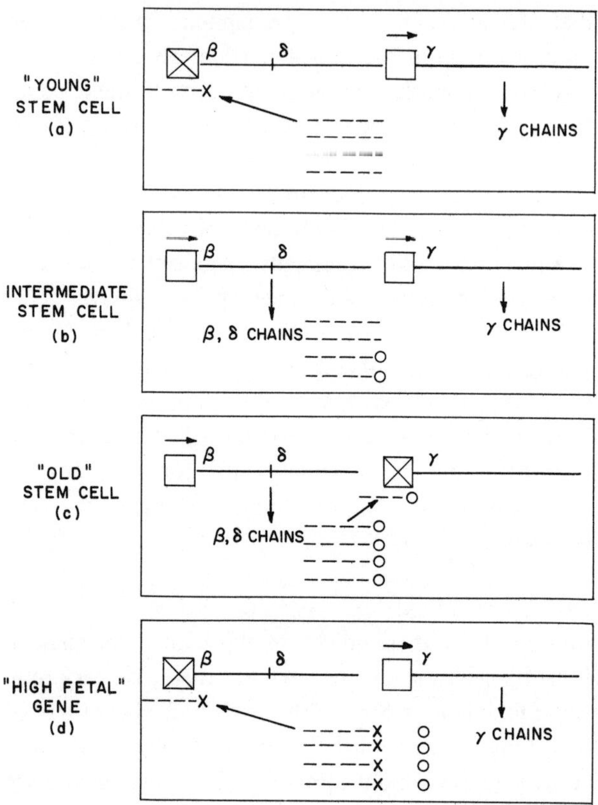

FIGURE 5-14. Model III for the mechanism which controls the switch from Hb-F to Hb-A production at the end of fetal life and in the "high fetal" gene condition

(a) Repressor type: -----
(b) Two repressor types: ---- and ----- 0, neither in sufficient concentration
(c) Repressor type: ----- 0
(d) Mutated repressor: ----- ✱ , which can no longer combine with 0, but still has the specificity to combine with the β/δ operator.

the β locus, there will be many blocked ribosomes in the cell incapable of contributing substantially to the production of hemoglobin. In this view the supply of ribosomes is limited and by blocking many of them the total production of hemoglobin in the cell is greatly reduced, which is what is observed. This is particularly so, if the β locus, like the α and the γ loci, produces a large number of β messengers (see chapter 4).

The δ structural gene, however, is perfectly normal and produces its usual normal δ messengers which, although few in number, produce normal δ chains and normal hemoglobin A_2 ($\alpha_2\delta_2$) in the usual amounts. In a heterozygote for a β chain thalassemia, the other β locus would be

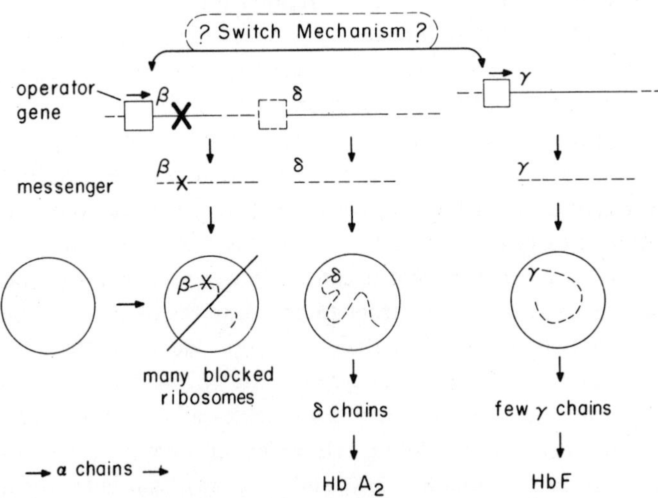

FIGURE 5-15. Model for the regulation of synthesis of hemoglobins A_2 and F in thalassemia major

normal and would lead to its quota of normal β peptide chains. However, two δ chain loci would be active in making δ chains, but only one β chain locus, leading to the observed increase in the ratio of hemoglobin A_2 ($\alpha_2\delta_2$) to A ($\alpha_2\beta_2$) in the heterozygote. Now turning back to the individual homozygous for a β chain thalassemia again, we know that fetal hemoglobin is produced in rather large amounts and therefore we know that the γ operator is turned on. Some γ messenger is therefore made and will occupy such ribosomes as are still available. The γ peptide chains are made and so is hemoglobin F ($\alpha_2\gamma_2$) as a result, but the compensation cannot be very effective, because so many of the limited supply of ribosomes are occupied and blocked by the defective

β messengers. As a result compensation for insufficient hemoglobin synthesis in thalassemia by the production of fetal hemoglobin is not very effective; the cells are still deficient in hemoglobin. In turn, in a manner unknown, this leads to destruction of these cells with consequent hemolytic anemia. More red cell production in the erythropoeitic tissues is called for and "younger" stem cells are used, according to Baglioni's ideas. Such cells are not repressed in the γ chain locus and are therefore capable of producing γ messengers and γ chains. In other words the mechanism by which there is even the observed amount of compensation with the production of fetal hemoglobin is that in thalassemia major cells, which are approximating the fetal type, are used. Of course in the alternative view, that β messenger RNA is itself the repressor for the γ operator (Figure 5-12), we could say that the defect already postulated to exist in the thalassemia β messenger RNA is of such a nature that it can no longer repress the γ operator. This second explanation is harder to accept in the case of a sickle-cell-thalassemia patient who has thalassemia of the interacting kind—β chain thalassemia. In this genotype ($\alpha^A/\alpha^A\ \beta^S/\beta^{Th}$) which is heterozygous for β chain thalassemia and for sickle-cell β chains there is also production of fetal hemoglobin. However, in these people many cells contain both hemoglobin S ($\alpha_2^A\beta_2^S$) and F ($\alpha_2^A\gamma_2^F$), that is to say their γ locus is derepressed. Here, however, two types of β chain messengers are presumed to be present, namely the β^S and the β^{Th} messenger RNA. There is no obvious reason why the former (β^S) messenger should not be quite capable of repressing the γ operator, if that is indeed one of the functions of normal β messengers, unless these repressors can only act in the same chromosome due to the chromosomal structure. One turns therefore more easily to the first explanation, namely that it is the blockage of protein synthesis which leads to the hemolytic anemia which leads in turn to the differentiation of a fetal type of cell in which the γ chain locus is not repressed.

THE "HIGH FETAL" GENE

In the very interesting genetic condition called the persistence of fetal hemoglobin (Edington and Lehmann, 1955) or the high fetal gene,

(Figure 5-12) we find that in the adult heterozygote there is a considerable amount of fetal hemoglobin made (up to 30 percent). There seem to be no clinical symptoms associated with this condition. There is also a heterozygous condition in which the high fetal gene occurs together with a sickle cell gene which is genetically linked. In such a heterozygote (of genotype $\alpha^A/\alpha^A\ \beta^{F\uparrow}/\beta^S$) there is about 70 percent of hemoglobin S, no hemoglobin A, but 30 percent of hemoglobin F. This is the proportion of sickle cell and of fetal hemoglobin which is found quite frequently in a sickle-cell homozygote in sickle-cell anemia. But whereas the sickle-cell homozygote is very ill indeed, these people heterozygous for hemoglobin S and the high fetal gene are not at all ill. Their condition compares with the sickle-cell heterozygote (A/S). There is in addition the case of a child (Wheeler and Krevans, 1961) who is homozygous for the high fetal gene and who has 100 percent of fetal hemoglobin in his blood. He is, however, perfectly healthy. The presence of only hemoglobin F is what one might expect in thalassemia major, but then this is a very severe disease whereas possession of the high fetal gene does not seem to cause any disease. One is struck by this difference between a thalassemia major individual who makes no β chains, that is no hemoglobin A, but who makes a large amount of fetal hemoglobin, on the one hand, and the person who is homozygous for the "high fetal" gene who also makes no hemoglobin A, but large amounts of fetal hemoglobin. In Figure 5-16 we see a scheme which seeks to explain the difference between thalassemia major and the "high fetal" homozygote, forgetting α chain production for the moment. This time we postulate a genetic defect in the switch mechanism such that the β operator cannot be switched on; however, the γ operator is permanently on. No β chain messenger is made at all and therefore the (limited) ribosomes are all available for occupancy by γ chain messenger RNA (and of course by α chain messenger RNA). The situation in the cells is therefore equivalent to that of a truly fetal cell, at least as far as the production of hemoglobin is concerned. Hemoglobin F synthesis can proceed efficiently and the cells contain a normal amount of hemoglobin. There is therefore no reason for a hemolytic anemia.

It is a curious fact that in the "high fetal" homozygote there is neither hemoglobin A nor hemoglobin A_2. In other words, neither β messenger RNA nor δ messenger RNA are made. If it is indeed true that one and the same operator and therefore the same switch mechanism controls the β and δ structural genes, then this is exactly what we would

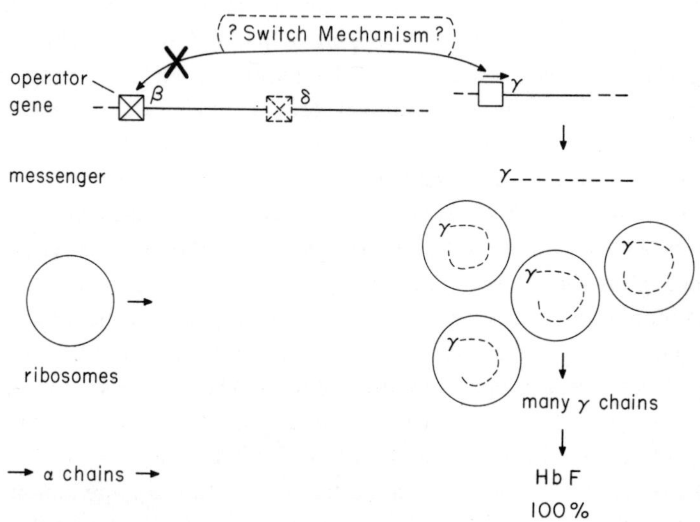

FIGURE 5-16. Model for the regulation of synthesis of hemoglobin F in the "high fetal" gene condition

expect to find in a situation where the switch is defective. Of course the genetic defect in the switch mechanism could take the form of a mutation affecting the repressor molecule in such a way that it is no longer capable of combining with the postulated hormone (Figure 5-14) to form the γ specific complex, but still represses the $\beta(+\delta)$ operator. This is a simpler postulate than another one which calls for a mutation in the β/δ operator, because then it would be difficult to see why the (unaltered) repressor should now derepress the γ locus. For this reason an altered repressor molecule is easier to accept (see also Figure 5-13).

Another explanation for the phenomenon of the "high fetal" gene which has been put forward by Conley (Bradley and Conley, 1960;

Herman and Conley, 1960) is that the basic defect is an overlapping deletion affecting both the β and the δ structural genes. In the present picture this deletion would result in no β or δ chain messenger being made. The rest of the scheme would be the same (Figure 5-12). At present we have no way of distinguishing between these two possibilities.

In a way, however, the heterozygote for the high fetal gene and for the sickle-cell gene is more difficult to explain. In his blood there is hemoglobin S and hemoglobin F with only, presumably, a small amount of hemoglobin A_2. Here one of the chromosomes containing the hemoglobin S mutation is of the adult type and if there is any repressor for γ chain loci involved then this should be present. In other words, it may well be in this individual that the γ chain locus belonging to the hemoglobin S chromosome is turned off whereas the γ chain locus linked with the high fetal gene is turned on. This would seem to rule out the role of diffusable repressor molecules unless we postulate that it is the structure of the chromosome itself which limits the diffusion of such repressing substances to just one chromosome.

If there is any justification for these speculations about the switch mechanisms, it is that they might stimulate some experiments. However, the explanation of these phenomena concerning the turning on and turning off of genes is so fundamental to any future understanding of the process of differentiation that even a speculation is worthwhile.

6

THE EVOLUTION OF THE HEMOGLOBINS

Evolution proceeds through natural selection acting on spontaneous variations. In examining this concept a little more closely, we find that we must postulate at least two different mechanisms.

Firstly, we need a device whereby the constancy of the genetic information is ensured. It is necessary to provide that succeeding generations should possess identical characteristics, to a first approximation. By identical characteristics we mean, at a molecular level, macromolecules and in particular protein molecules of a chemical structure identical with those found in the parent, as well as identical patterns of differentiation. Such a mechanism of stability can easily be provided by the action of DNA acting in its capacity as a store and conveyor of information required for the synthesis of the body constituents. In particular the conservative nature of DNA replication and the way in which DNA hands on its message to the protein synthesizing machinery will ensure that the primary structure of the all-important protein molecules will be identical.

Secondly, we need a different mechanism which allows for the production of the variations in an organism on which the forces of natural selection can act. For example, the mutations in the genetic material which result in inherited changes in the primary structure of proteins form such a mechanism. The simplest examples of such mutations are the so-called point mutations, which seem to result in the substitution of individual amino acid residues in proteins by different amino acid residues. Such a change leads sometimes to a distinct change in the physical properties of the affected protein and consequently to an alteration in the physiological behavior of that protein. Should the change be beneficial to the animal, then this particular variation will be favored by natural selection; it will be perpetuated and will perhaps become predominant. It is well to remember that a particular amino acid alteration in a protein, to be selected favorably, must ultimately produce an increase in the number of progency of its possessor.

Other types of mutation will certainly occur, most of them deleterious; those will eventually be eliminated. However, even a deleterious mutation might prove beneficial to its possessor, if it should happen that the environment should change in such a direction that the mutation is now no longer deleterious, but under the new conditions is advantageous. As well as the so-called point mutations, other inherited variations of protein structure can be envisaged, such as the deletion of genetic material which would result in the loss of some amino acid sequences of a peptide chain. Alternatively, the addition of genetic material could occur with its consequent addition of amino acid sequences to the peptide chain.

From the point of view of the evolutionary argument, none of the mutations mentioned in Figure 3-17 would be straightforward cases of an advantageous variation, since they either have no advantage or are deleterious. On the other hand, those which are found with high frequency must possess some advantage for an individual carrier in order to explain a high frequency, resulting in a situation of balanced polymorphism. We see for example in hemoglobin S, how changes in the information controlling the primary structure of a protein can lead to pronounced alterations in the physiological behavior of the resulting protein molecule. We can imagine by an extension of these arguments that the kind of variability needed for the evolutionary development of a protein might be of this general type where amino acid substitutions produce changes which ultimately result in a better and more advantageous hemoglobin molecule. At the same time there are undoubtedly always amino acid substitutions in the less important part of the protein molecule, so that we can say that in the course of evolution the structure of a particular protein will fluctuate around a certain "structural optimum." There will be changes in the primary structure of this protein which are of no particular selective advantage or disadvantage and which occur spontaneously and are not necessarily eliminated quickly. In other words, it is not necessary to postulate that every amino acid difference between a higher and a lower vertebrate necessarily implies that in this particular region of the peptide chain the higher organism has a more advantageous structure. We may be looking merely at these spontaneous fluctuations in protein structure produced by mutations.

Let us turn now to a more detailed consideration of these principles in the case of the proteins hemoglobin and myoglobin. Hemoglobin is a particularly useful model for examining the mechanism of evolution of a protein; so much is known about its chemistry and about its mutability, and it is also universally found in the vertebrate phylum. Hemoglobin shows promise of forming one day a coherent evolutionary story, but even today we can use it to illustrate the principles which we have just enumerated.

GENETIC CONTROL OF PRIMARY, SECONDARY, AND TERTIARY PROTEIN STRUCTURE

In Kendrew's (1961) three-dimensional model of the related protein myoglobin we are impressed by the complexity of such a protein molecule. In the peptide chain of myoglobin, which is some hundred and forty amino acids long, the sequence of these amino acids is quite definite and unique. Presumably it is the DNA information mechanism which is responsible for the production of such a complex molecule with such exactness. The intricate folding which is apparent in this model is also unique and to a large extent is thought to be a consequence of the particular primary structure of this protein. The insertion of the heme group in its correct place is assured by the accurately determined structure of the protein surface. All this is an excellent example of the precise control exercised by the conservative DNA information carrying mechanism (and also of the tremendous achievement of the x-ray crystallographers!).

In Perutz's model (Perutz *et al.*, 1960; Perutz, 1962) of horse hemoglobin we are also impressed by the intricate and precise coiling of the four peptide chains which make up this molecule, although here we see only the outlines of the chains, not the detailed amino acid sequences. The two α peptide chains are identical and symmetrically arranged around the central axis. The two identical β chains are also symmetrically arranged around the same axis. Again, the genetic information needed for making such a complex protein molecule is precise and exact. In the case of hemoglobin even more genetic information is required than for some other proteins, because this is a complex protein consisting of four peptide chains and four iron-porphyrin complexes, the heme groups. The four heme groups are made in the cell by a series of enzymes; these enzymes are themselves proteins and require for their functioning that they be accurately made by their own particular genes. All in all, in order to produce the hemoglobin molecule, precise genetic information is needed to ensure the synthesis of the correct α and β peptide chains and in addition the production of the various enzymes involved in the synthesis of heme.

Inherent in all our arguments is the assumption that the amino acid sequence of the protein—its primary structure—determines the coiling of the peptide chains and thereby the chemical nature of the surface of the protein to which its most important biochemical properties are due. This assumption is likely to be true for a small protein up to a molecular weight of, say 20,000, whether or not the final structure is stabilized by disulfide bridges. Haber and Anfinsen (unpublished) have shown the effect of tyrosine-tyrosine interactions in promoting the refolding and reactivation of reduced pancreatic ribonuclease. Their finding supports the idea that primary structure determines folding.

A simple mechanism for folding becomes increasingly unlikely with increasing molecular weight and complexity, since a large molecule has probably a number of energetically equivalent tertiary structures; these, however, may be by no means equivalent in their biological specificity. And how is it determined which of these configurations will be favored? It may very well depend on the interaction of the folding chain with some other protein, itself genetically determined, or with some simple substrate, present due to the action of (genetically determined) enzymes. Thus rather subtle interactions are possible.

PLEIOTROPISM

The primary alteration in a mutated protein may affect not only that protein, but also others with which it is interacting. Genetically, the simultaneous expression of a single mutation as a bouquet of effects is well known as "pleiotropism." We can see a possible molecular mechanism for pleiotropism in the interactions of a single mutated protein with a number of different biochemical systems.

At the level of the first protein product of the gene, pleiotropism probably does not exist unless the mutated protein, *by virtue of its mutation*, folds in two or more different ways or forms two or more species of carbohydrate derivative, etc. It seems likely, on the other hand, that most cases of genetic pleiotropism will be explained as a single enzyme or protein defect leading to two or more manifestations, because of interaction with different biochemical systems. A class of truly pleiotropic molecules are groups of mutated hemoglobins, such as hemoglobins $D_{\text{St. Louis}}$ $(\alpha_2^{\text{St. L.}}\ \beta_2^{\text{A}})$ and $F_{\text{St. Louis}}$ $(\alpha_2^{\text{St. L.}}\ \gamma_2^{\text{F}})$ or hemoglobins Norfolk $(\alpha_2^{\text{Norf}}\ \beta_2^{\text{A}})$ and Norfolk$_2$ $(\alpha_2^{\text{Norf}}\ \delta_2^{\text{A}_2})$, where a single α chain mutation leads to two or three distinct hemoglobin variants. The argument is good so long as one considers the whole hemoglobin molecule as the unit, rather than either α or β peptide chain.

The tendency in the field of "molecular genetics" has been to concentrate on exploring very simple experimental systems in order to illustrate clearly some general principle. We will rapidly have to become more sophisticated, however, if we want to understand the molecular basis of evolution or molecular disease, fundamentally similar phenomena. We need think only of the recent work on complementation (Fincham, 1960) or the current discussion of the different forms of thalassemia (Ingram and Stretton, 1959; Itano and Pauling, 1961; Rucknagel and Neel, 1961).

VERTEBRATE HEMOGLOBINS

A great deal of experimental work is being done in comparing the structural aspects of the vertebrate hemoglobins with the human hemoglobin (see review in Gratzer and Allison, 1960). One fundamental point which has emerged is that the hemoglobins of the vertebrates are all remarkably similar, not only in the sense that they are proteins with the same type of heme group attached to them, but also in the sense that they are similar in the overall architecture of the molecule. Right down to the cartilagenous fishes, the vertebrate hemoglobins which have been studied contain four peptide chains of molecular weight 17,000 and they can all be expressed by a formula such as $\alpha_2\beta_2$. Below the fishes, the hemoglobins are different. The hemoglobin of the lamprey is peculiar in consisting of a single polypeptide chain of molecular weight 17,000. The hagfish hemoglobin appears to be similar, or possibly a dimer of 34,000 molecular weight.

Many of the vertebrate hemoglobins have not only one hemoglobin component but two, a situation which is very reminiscent of the human, where we have hemoglobin A and hemoglobin A_2. It has become clear from the work being done by Schweet (1962) and by Muller (1961) that in some of the animals which do have multiple hemoglobins the two types share one subunit, and that they may be written as $\alpha_2\beta_2$ and $\alpha_2\delta_2$. It looks as if in the course of evolution the architecture of this important molecule had reached a certain degree of perfection early on and from then on had evolved in a conservative fashion. We mean by this that the hemoglobin was subject to variations of the type which is illustrated by the amino acid substitutions in the abnormal hemoglobins (Figure 3-17, for example) and subject also to other types of variation. The overriding consideration, however, seems to be that the function of this molecule has to remain that of a hemoglobin. It may well be that the "reason" for a four subunit structure is that this provides a mechanism for increasing the efficiency of the physiological functioning of the whole molecule by the so-called "interaction" of the four heme groups. It is this heme-heme interaction of a vertebrate hemoglobin which makes it such an efficient oxygen carrier. A plot of the degree of oxygenation of the hemoglobin molecules against the partial pressure of oxygen is sigmoid in shape, illustrating the ability of hemoglobin to take up oxygen rapidly in the lungs and to deoxygenate easily in the tissues. Provided these aspects of the molecular structure are preserved, the rest, or rather the amino acid sequences determining the rest of the structure, could change in the course of evolution.

It is interesting to consider and to compare hemoglobin with other closely related proteins, for example the myoglobins, which are one-chain molecules. The function of myoglobin in the muscle is to store oxygen and therefore it also has the ability to combine reversibly with oxygen. Myoglobin has obvious structural relationships in terms of amino acid sequence to hemoglobin (Watson and Kendrew, 1961) but it is a different branch of the same family. There are undoubtedly a few similarities in structure between myoglobins and hemoglobins of the same species, but recently Hill (unpublished) has shown that the chemical structure of human myoglobin is more like that of sperm whale myoglobin than it is like human hemoglobin. It seems that it is much more important for this protein to be a myoglobin with the structural characteristics which make it a myoglobin than that it should be a human protein.

The existence of the multiple hemoglobins in humans and animals is a striking fact which is still difficult to understand. Human hemoglobin A_2 is interesting from a genetic point of view, but it is difficult to see a definite physiological role for it, since it amounts to only 2.5 percent of the total hemoglobin content. Is it a hemoglobin on its way out from an evolutionary point of view? Is it a hemoglobin eventually destined to replace hemoglobin A? Then how can it make its presence felt in view of the small amount present? It has been suggested (Gluecksohn-Waelsch, 1960) that the possession of multiple hemoglobins acts as a buffer against mutational change, since a deleterious effect in one form of hemoglobin may be compensated for by the production of the other type.

HOMOLOGY BETWEEN α AND β PEPTIDE CHAINS

When examining the complete amino acid sequences of the α and β peptide chains of adult human hemoglobin (Figure 2-5), one is immediately struck by the great degree of homology which exists between these two peptide chains, since almost 40 amino acid residues (out of 141) are identical. It is this kind of chemical evidence which leads one to postulate that the α and β chains of human hemoglobin A are perhaps derived from a common ancestor (Itano, 1957; Gratzer and Allison, 1960; Ingram, 1961; Braunitzer *et al.*, 1961b; Zuckerkandl and Pauling, 1962). In order to show this high degree of homology

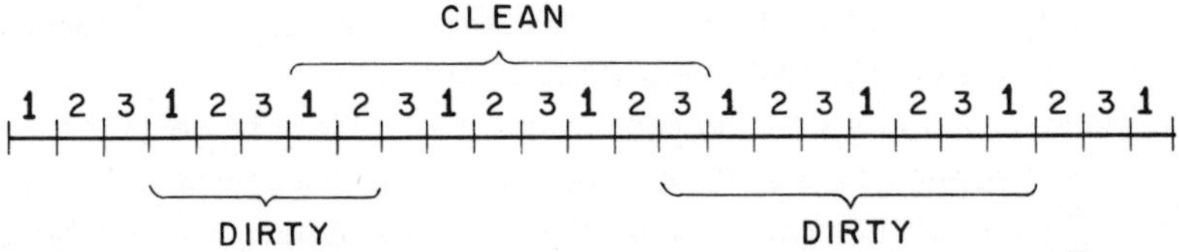

FIGURE 6-1. Diagrammatic representation of the "triplet code" of DNA

The extent of "clean" and "dirty" deletions of genetic material is indicated. (Ingram, 1962.)

between α and β chains placed side by side, it is necessary to introduce apparent "gaps" in the amino acid sequences at a few places (Braunitzer *et al.*, 1961). These are, of course, not gaps in covalent structure, but an artifact of the illustration, since the amino acids are joined across them in the usual way by peptide bonds. It seems as if a few amino acid sequences had been deleted in the course of evolution, in the course of divergence from a common ancestor. On the other hand, the amino acids found opposite to these "gaps" may be due to the addition of genetic material.

If we believe that the deoxyribonucleic acid (DNA) of the genetic material carries a code for the specific hemoglobin sequence, then we must distinguish between two kinds of deletion: *clean deletions* of DNA which extend exactly from the beginning of one coding unit to the end of the same or some following coding unit (Figure 6-1); thus, no "nonsense" is produced; and *dirty deletions* of DNA which start and/or finish within coding units (see Ingram, 1962). These latter may leave "nonsense" at either end which might lead to a break in the peptide chain or to an interruption of protein synthesis. Alternatively, by a mechanism similar to that proposed by Crick *et al.* (1961), for certain forms of mutagenesis, the code subsequent to the dirty deletion might read entirely differently, having now a new starting point. In this latter case, the affected portion of the peptide chain would be very strange and not recognizably hemoglobin. On both counts, dirty deletions would be harmful and therefore eliminated in the course of evolution. The "gaps" we see in the human hemoglobin chains of today are likely to derive from clean deletions, since there are many homologous amino acid sequences both before and after the "gaps."

What of additions to the genetic material leading to an increased length of peptide chain? We cannot point to any biochemical illustrations of this phenomenon among the abnormal human hemoglobins, or anywhere else, but we might equally well interpret the "gaps" in Braunitzer's hemoglobin chains as "additions" of amino acids in the homologous chain. The α and β chains of human hemoglobin are unequal in length (141 and 146 residues), yet similar in amino acid sequence at each end. This state of affairs could have arisen either by a succession of deletions or by the addition of genetic material within the gene. If the former explanation were the correct one, we would deduce that the mode of action of evolution is to change and shorten chains and that the ancestral chains were all longer than their modern counterparts; this is an unlikely situation. It is more probable that additions, clean additions, also occurred.

We can also deduce that certain regions of the peptide chain should not be altered in the course of divergence and evolution; they are presumably needed to maintain the correct folding of these chains and thereby the proper functioning of the molecule. There is some evidence that the so-called "basic center" of the hemoglobin peptide chains (α56 – 62, β61 – 67 in the human) is very similar in structure in the cow, horse, sheep, rabbit, and goat hemoglobins (Braunitzer *et al.*, 1961; Muller, 1961; Zuckerkandl and Pauling, 1962; Naughton and Dintzis, 1962). Equally, certain other sites on the peptide chain can be altered without affecting too much the final functioning of the molecule.

HOMOLOGY BETWEEN β, γ, AND δ CHAINS

Next we turn to a consideration of the β and γ peptide chain sequences of human adult ($\alpha_2\beta_2$) and human fetal ($\alpha_2\gamma_2$) hemoglobin (Schroeder *et al.*, 1962). The degree of homology between the β and the γ peptide chains (Figure 5-4) is even more striking than the homology between α and β. The two chains are of equal length (146 residues) and two thirds of the amino acid sequences are identical. This degree of homology would lead one to believe—in evolutionary terms—that the β and γ peptide chains diverged at a later stage.

The relationship between the β and δ peptide chains is closest of all (Figure 4-3; Ingram and Stretton, 1961, 1962), since only 7 – 8 single amino acid substitutions have appeared so far. Moreover, the N-terminal and C-terminal sequences are identical and it is highly probable that the overall chain lengths are the same (Stretton, unpublished). For this reason we assume that the β and δ chains have diverged very recently in evolutionary history. Zuckerkandl and Pauling (1962) estimate this event to have taken place some 44 million years ago, at the time of the origin of the primates.

POSTULATES FOR THE EVOLUTIONARY SCHEME

The great similarity which characterizes most vertebrate hemoglobins suggest that we are studying that aspect of the evolution of a particular protein molecule which is concerned with the detailed development of an already well-defined molecule. It is true that the hemoglobin quadruples its size during this evolution (if we include the lamprey hemoglobin), but the change is due to the aggregation of four fairly similar protein subunits (peptide chains), rather than to an actual lengthening of a molecule. In the evolutionary scheme to be discussed it is suggested that the increase in complexity, and in diversity, of the hemoglobins is an illustration of a more general process of gene evolution which results in an increase of the number of genes.

The following postulates are used in developing a scheme for the evolution of the hemoglobin genes.

(1) Mutations of a gene result in either single or multiple amino acid substitutions in the peptide chain which that gene controls, in inversions

of part of the amino acid sequence, in deletions or additions, or in a combination of these possibilities. The new hemoglobin peptide chains produced by such mutations are then either favored or discarded in the course of natural selection.

(2) At several points in the course of evolution a gene for a particular hemoglobin peptide chain has undergone duplication, followed by, or simultaneous with, translocation of the duplicated gene. The two initially equivalent genes have then evolved independently, governed by the selective pressure of their environment on their protein products. Such mechanisms have been postulated previously (Bridges, 1936; Lewis, 1951); in particular, the role of gene duplication in evolution has been discussed by Stephens (1951). His conclusion was that the case for duplication as an important factor in evolution was neither proved nor disproved. It seems likely that the α and β genes are located on different chromosomes, since they segregate independently, whereas β and δ genes appear to be linked (Ceppellini, 1959). We know nothing of the location of the γ genes as yet, since we have no mutants of that chain.

SCHEME FOR THE EVOLUTION OF THE HEMOGLOBIN GENES

In Figure 6-2 an evolutionary scheme for the hemoglobin genes is proposed (Ingram, 1961b) in which the origins of the four hemoglobin genes and of the obviously related myoglobin gene are traced to a common ancestor, using postulate (2). At the four points indicated in Figure 6-2, gene duplications led ultimately to independent genes. In this scheme, the chains which are most different, the myoglobin peptide chains, are put farthest apart and the genes controlling chains which are very closely related, as β and δ, are put most closely together. There is no obvious reason for putting the γ chain before the β chain in development, except that one generally regards the fetal proteins, or fetal morphological features, as being more primitive.

In this connection it may be worth pointing out, that although in the embryonic development of an advanced vertebrate there seem to be stages which recapitulate the evolution of the vertebrate phylum, this does not necessarily imply that at that stage the genes producing, for example, gill-like structures are really the same genes which produce the corresponding structures in fishes. It may merely mean that gill-like structures are produced from human proteins and other human macromolecules and that it is the mechanism which controls *differentiation* of the human embryo which still contains some information similar to the primitive information which used to control the differentiation of the fish embryo.

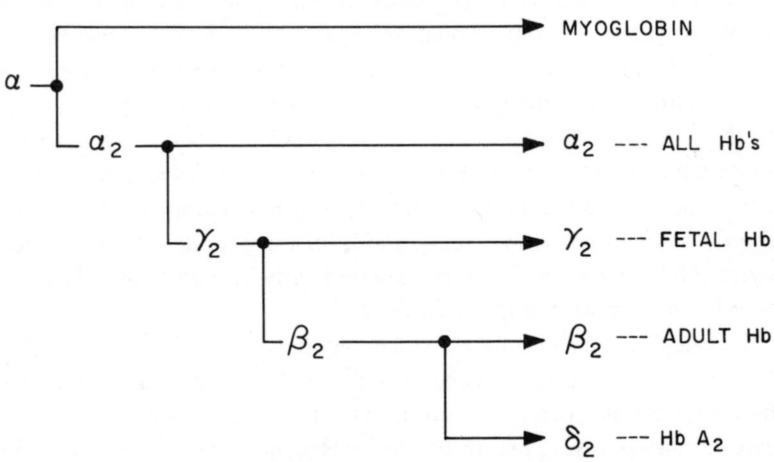

FIGURE 6-2. Evolution of the hemoglobin chains
The point in time of a gene duplication is indicated by a solid black circle.

We might suppose that originally the hemoglobin molecule was rather like the present-day myoglobin molecule, that is, that it had a single peptide chain with a single heme group and therefore it could not show heme-heme interaction. The size of this molecule might vary, but eventually it was stabilized at approximately 17,000 molecular weight.

At this stage of evolution, presumably earlier than the teleost fishes, the heme protein inside the muscle cells is assumed to be the same as that in the circulation. The muscle heme protein became myoglobin in the course of evolution; it retained a molecular weight of 17,000 and a complexity of only one heme group and one peptide chain per molecule. It was, of course, still subject to mutational changes, as can be seen from the fact that its present-day amino acid composition and sequence in a given animal often differs considerably from that of any of the analogous hemoglobin chains (Rossi-Fanelli *et al.*, 1955). For example, human myoglobin contains isoleucine, but no cysteine, whereas the reverse is true of human adult hemoglobin.

On the other hand, one can foresee limits to the kind of mutations which would be tolerated. The x-ray studies of Kendrew and of Perutz show that the three-dimensional arrangement of chains in myoglobin and the hemoglobin subunits (also of 17,000 molecular weight) are remarkably similar, though not identical. This statement applies also to the two kinds of subunits found in hemoglobin itself. Presumably, mutational alterations in the course of evolution which would drastically affect the three-dimensional structure were not tolerated. Such considerations imply that the configuration of the peptide chains in myoglobin and hemoglobin became stabilized early in evolutionary history, at least in its most important features.

During the evolution of the first hemoglobin chain—the α chain in this scheme—there occurred a gene duplication followed or accompanied by translocation. From now on the two duplicate α chain genes could evolve independently, one to become the modern myoglobin gene, the other to become the α chain gene of present-day hemoglobin. Eventually, according to the scheme, the α chain gene would evolve in such a way that its product, the α chain, had the property of dimerization in solution to form α_2 molecules. Such a property would be favored strongly, if it entailed, in addition, the possibility of heme-heme interaction between the two heme groups of the new dimer molecule and therefore the possibility of more efficient oxygenation and deoxygenation. Once produced, such a mutation is unlikely to be lost in the further evolution of hemoglobin.

We might next postulate that the genes of the α chains duplicated again. After this gene duplication two types of dimer—α_2 and γ_2—would evolve side by side. Sooner or later, these chains would have evolved sufficiently to be able to form tetramers with even greater selective advantage, because of the increased heme-heme interaction likely to be found in such tetramers. The characteristics of the genes responsible for the ability of the chains to form tetramers would certainly be fixed from then on. This stage of hemoglobin evolution seems to have been reached already in some teleost fishes, because they already possess a four-chain hemoglobin (see in Gratzer and Allison, 1960).

The third gene duplication and translocation is pictured as occurring with the γ chain gene, giving rise to a new γ gene destined to evolve into the β chain gene. At this gene duplication the property of forming tetramers is already firmly established. The new gene can develop along its own lines to provide a hemoglobin tetramer, $\alpha_2\beta_2$, particularly adapted for the adult body. On the other hand, the old γ chain continues to develop and to provide half the molecule of the fetal hemoglobin ($\alpha_2\gamma_2$). It is the γ chain gene, rather than the α chain gene, which is said to duplicate here, because the γ chain dimers, γ_2, have already the necessary complementariness for forming tetramers with α_2. This complementariness will be automatically a property of the product of the new gene. In addition, β and γ chains are more closely related to one another than either is related to the α chain. Therefore we might consider them to have diverged at a later stage.

At this point in evolution, three independent genes—α, β, γ—are assumed to be present, each one capable of forming chains which dimerize and which aggregate to the tetramers $\alpha_2\beta_2$ or $\alpha_2\gamma_2$. Heme-heme interaction is strongly present in the tetramers. Such a situation has an important effect on the further evolution of the α chain. This chain, or rather its dimer, α_2, is required to fit with two different partners, β_2 and γ_2. As a result, less variation is allowed to the α chain; it has become "conservative." Perhaps such conservatism is in part responsible for the apparently universal presence of α chains beginning with val-leu- in the hemoglobins of the higher vertebrates from teleosts on. There is an alternative explanation for the apparently greater stability of the α genes; this gene controls also the fetal hemoglobin and therefore may not undergo extensive mutational alterations, since the fetus or larva is a much more delicate organism. The very fact that any alteration in the α chain gene, and therefore in the α chain, seems to affect all types of hemoglobin may be sufficient to explain the apparent "conservatism." However, the "conservatism" of the α chain may be more apparent than real and may be confined to the N-terminal sequence of the chain. There is no *a priori* reason why different parts of a molecule as complex as a protein should develop at the same rate. The difference in apparent stability between the α chain and the other could, of course, be no more than what would be expected as normal variation. It will be interesting to see just how similar the val-leu- chains of different vertebrates are.

At the fourth and last gene duplication in the scheme we suppose that it is the β gene which is duplicated, leading to the δ chain genes controlling the δ chains of hemoglobin A_2. The origin of this δ chain is placed near the end of the evolutionary scheme, because of its great chemical similarity to the β chain. Furthermore, the presence of a hemoglobin A_2-like component seems to be confined to the higher primates (Kunkel *et al.*, 1957). In this view, hemoglobin A_2 is a new hemoglobin rather than an archaic one, as has often been supposed. It has been reported to have a higher affinity for oxygen (Meyering *et al.*, 1960), and perhaps it is a more efficient hemoglobin, destined to replace eventually $\alpha_2\beta_2$. Since there is genetic evidence that the genes for δ and for β chains are linked, perhaps the process of translocation of the new δ gene has not yet occurred.

Where does the lamprey fit into this scheme? One form, Petromyzon planeri, has two larval and two (different) adult hemoglobins (Adinolfi *et al.*, 1959). The molecular weight of the adult mixture is given as 17,000. Perhaps these lamprey hemoglobins are the result of an independent evolutionary scheme similar to the one discussed here, but which has never included the mutations which led to the formation of dimers and tetramers. On the other hand, some features of the fingerprint patterns of tryptic digests of the larval and adult lamprey hemoglobins show definite resemblances (Siniscalco, unpublished), as would be expected on the basis of a common ancestor. We might regard the lampreys as having branched off before or just after the first gene duplication in the scheme of Figure 6-2. Unfortunately, nothing seems to be known about the presence or absence of a separate myoglobin in the lampreys.

It has been suggested that the four genes controlling the four chains might have evolved from four unrelated genes which originally controlled the synthesis of quite unrelated proteins; thus there would have been no increase in the total number of genes. By a process of parallel evolution—successive and independent mutations—each of these four genes eventually changed so that it made one of the hemoglobin peptide chains. The last stages of evolution, when pairs of genes were involved in producing parts of a complex molecule, must then be called on to produce similarity in chemical structure and in configuration. It is easy to conceive of a selective mechanism which would favor changes in various members of a molecular aggregate, such that the members might fit together better. However, it is hard to think of such a mechanism also selecting for chemical and structural similarity of the monomers. In addition, the ability to dimerize would have to arise *de novo* four times, an unlikely situation. Although we cannot at the moment completely reject the idea of parallel evolution of the four hemoglobin genes from unrelated genes, it is not a very appealing one.

CHEMICAL AND EVOLUTIONARY RELATIONSHIP BETWEEN THE CHAINS

How many mutational steps occurred between the original α gene and the present-day human α gene? Or between the original α gene and the human β gene? It is more meaningful, perhaps, to ask how many mutational events as a minimum might separate the present-day human α and β genes. Out of 141 amino acids, we know from the sequences that 85 are different. This gives a *minimum* of 85 mutations of the kind effecting single amino acid substitutions.

It is generally believed that the evolution of the vertebrates began some 5×10^8 years ago. Let us assume a mean generation life of 5 years among the vertebrates, which implies some 10^8 generations for the evolution of vertebrate hemoglobins. A generally acceptable mutation rate per generation is 10^{-5}–10^{-6}, which leads to a figure of 100–1,000 mutations in the evolutionary history of a vertebrate hemoglobin. This figure, which is itself a minimum one, is considerably higher than the (minimum) number of mutations which appear to distinguish α chains from β chains or α chains from γ chains.

The only conclusion which can be drawn from such a calculation is that a more than sufficient number of mutational events has passed in the history of the vertebrates to account for present-day differences between the various parts of the hemoglobin molecule in the human species (Zuckerkandl and Pauling, 1962).

In this connection it is interesting to note that Zuckerkandl and Schroeder (1961) find that the α chains of gorilla hemoglobin differ from human α chains by perhaps no more than two amino acid residues; an aspartic acid replaces glutamic acid and possibly a serine residue is missing in the gorilla α chain. Since these findings are based on total amino acid analyses of the separated chain, it remains to be seen whether other differences exist in the sequences of these chains. They also report that the gorilla β chain has a lysine residue replacing an arginine. None of these substitutions affects the charge on the molecule and as a result human and gorilla hemoglobin have the same electrophoretic mobilities.

Fingerprints of hemoglobins from other mammals (Muller, 1961) are recognizable as "hemoglobin." The degree of similarity in fingerprints between the mammalian hemoglobins is great, while chicken hemoglobin shows considerable differences.

Recently, Zuckerkandl *et al.* (1960) have shown that fingerprints of hemoglobin from the gorilla and the chimpanzee are indistinguishable from those of human hemoglobin. A greater number of differing peptide spots are observed in the less closely related orangutan and rhesus monkey. As one moves away from the primates, the differences in fingerprint patterns increase until one finds that fish hemoglobins give radically different fingerprints. In spite of such differences in behavior of the peptides, there might still be similarites of sequence between the points of difference. These extraordinarily interesting findings give added proof of the validity of using a chemical study of vertebrate hemoglobins to discover evolutionary relationships.

BIBLIOGRAPHY

Adinolfi, M. *et al.* [G. Chieffi and M. Siniscalco]. 1959. Haemoglobin pattern of the cyclostome Petromyzon planeri during the course of development. Nature, London, 184: 1325.

Adinolfi, M. *et al.* [L. Bernini, B. Latte, A. Motulsky, and M. Siniscalco]. 1961. The distribution of G6PD-deficiency and of thalassemia in Italy and its relationship to malaria. Second Int. Conf. of Human Genetics, Rome, Abstract 123. Publ. Excerpta Medica, Amsterdam.

Ager, J. A. M., and H. Lehmann. 1958. Observations on some "fast" haemoglobins: K, J, N and "Bart's". Brit. Med. J., 1: 929.

Ager, J. A. M. *et al.* [H. Lehmann and F. Vella]. 1958. Haemoglobin "Norfolk": a new haemoglobin found in an english family. Brit. Med. J. 2: 539.

Allen, D. W., and J. H. Jandl. 1960. Factors influencing relative rates of synthesis of adult and fetal hemoglobin *in vitro*. J. Clin. Invest., 39: 1107.

Allison, A. C. 1954. Protection afforded by sickle-cell trait against subtertian malarial infection. Brit. Med. J., 1: 290.

Allison, A. C. 1956. Sickle cells and evolution. Sci. American, August, p. 87.

Allison, A. C. 1957. Exp. Parasitol., 6: 418.

Allison, A. C. *et al.* [B. S. Blumberg and A. Reep]. 1958. Haptoglobin types in British, Spanish Basque and Nigerian African populations. Nature, London, 181: 824.

Atwater, J. *et al.* [I. R. Schwartz and C. M. Tocantins]. 1960. A variety of human hemoglobin with four distinct electrophoretic components. Blood, 15: 901.

Baglioni, C. 1961. An improved method for the fingerprinting of human haemoglobin. Biochim et Biophys. Acta, 48: 392.

Baglioni, C. 1962a. Correlations between genetics and chemistry of human haemoglobins. In Progress in Molecular Genetics. (Ed. H. Taylor), New York, Academic Press.

Baglioni, C. 1962b. Abnormal human haemoglobins. VIII. Biochim. et Biophys. Acta, 59: 437.

Baglioni, C. 1962c. A chemical study of hemoglobin Norfolk. J. Biol. Chem., 237: 69.

Baglioni, C., and V. M Ingram. 1961. Four adult haemoglobin types in one person. Nature, London, 189: 465.

Baglioni, C. *et al.* [V. M. Ingram and E. Sullivan]. 1961. Genetic control of foetal and adult human haemoglobin. Nature, London, 189: 467.

Bannerman, R. M. 1961. Thalassemia. New York, Grune and Stratton.

Barnabas, J., and C. J. Muller. 1962. Haemoglobin $\text{Lepore}_{\text{Hollandia}}$. Nature, London, 194: 931.

Beadle, G. W., and E. L. Tatum. 1941. Genetic control of biochemical reactions in Neurospora. Pro. Nat. Acad. Sci. U.S., 27: 499.

Beet, E. A. 1949. The genetics of the sickle-cell trait in a Bantu tribe. Annals of Eugenics, 14: 279.

Benzer, S., and B. Weisblum. 1961. On the species specificity of acceptor RNA and attachment enzymes. Pro. Nat. Acad. Sci. U.S., 47: 1149.

Benzer, S. *et al.* [V. M. Ingram and H. Lehmann]. 1958. Three varieties of human haemoglobin D. Nature, London, 182: 852.

Berg, P. 1961. Specificity in protein synthesis. Ann. Rev. of Biochem., 30: 293.

Betke, K. 1958. Hämoglobinanomalien. Schweiz. med. Wochschr., 88: 1005.

Beutler, E. *et al.* [R. J. Dern and C. L. Flanagan]. 1955. Effect of sickle-cell trait on resistance to malaria. Brit. Med. J., 1: 1189.

Bianco, L. *et al.* [G. Montalenti, E. Silvestroni, and M. Siniscalco]. 1952. Further data on genetics of microcythaemia or thalassemia minor and Cooley's disease or thalassemia major. Annals of Eugenics, 16: 299.

Boulard, C. *et al.* [A. Cosset, F. Destaing, A. Duzer, J. H. P. Jonxis, C. J. Muller, and A. Portier]. 1961. Hb I trait in an Algerian muselman family, presenting two abnormal components. Blood, 18: 750.

Bowman, B., and V. M. Ingram. 1962. Abnormal human haemoglobins. VII. Biochim. et Biophys. Acta, 53: 569.

Bradley, T. B., and C. L. Conley. 1960. Trans. Assoc. Am. Physicians, 73: 72.

Braunitzer, G., and V. Rudloff. 1962. Die Hämoglobine. Deut. med. Wochschr., 87: 959.

Braunitzer, G. *et al.* [B. Liebold, R. Müller, and V. Rudloff]. 1960. Der homologe chemische Aufbau der Peptidketten in Humanhämoglobin A. Hoppe-Seyler's Z. physiol. Chem., 320: 171.

Braunitzer, G. *et al.* [R. Gehring-Müller, N. Hilschmann, K. Hilse, G. Hobam, V. Rudloff, and B. Wittmann-Liebold]. 1961a. Die Konstitution des normalen adulten Humanhämoglobins. Hoppe-Seyler's Z. physiol. Chem., 325: 283.

Braunitzer, G. *et al.* [N. Hilschmann, V. Rudloff, K. Hilse, B. Liebold, and

R. Müller]. 1961b. The haemoglobin particles—chemical and genetic aspects of their structure. Nature, London, 190: 480.

Brenner, S., F. Jacob, and M. Meselson. 1961. An unstable intermediate carrying information from genes to ribosomes for protein synthesis. Nature, London, 190: 576.

Bridges, C. B. 1936. The bar "gene": a duplication. Science, 83: 210.

Cabannes, R., and A. Portier. 1959. *In* Abnormal Haemoglobins. (Eds. J. H. P. Jonxis and J. F. Delafresnaye), Oxford, Blackwell, p. 61.

Ceppellini, R. 1959a. Acta Genet. Med. et Gemellol., 8: 47.

Ceppellini, R. 1959b. Biochemistry of Human Genetics. *In* Ciba Foundation Symp. (Eds. G. E. W. Wolstenholme and C. M. O'Connor), London, Churchill, p. 133.

Chernoff, A. I. 1959. The distribution of the thalassemia gene: a historical review. Blood, 14: 899.

Connell, G. E. *et al.* [G. H. Dixon and O. Smithies]. 1962. Subdivision of the three common haptoglobin types based on "hidden" differences. Nature, London, 193: 505.

Cook, C. D. *et al.* [H. R. Brodie and D. W. Allen]. 1957. Measurement of fetal hemoglobin in newborn infants. Pediatrics, 20: 272.

Crick, F. H. C. *et al.* [L. Barnett, S. Brenner, and R. J. Watts-Tobin]. 1961. General nature of the genetic code for proteins. Nature, London, 192: 1227.

Dintzis, H. M. 1961. Assembly of the peptide chains of hemoglobin. Pro. Nat. Acad. Sci. U.S., 47: 247.

Dreyer, W. 1960. Brookhaven Symp. in Biology, 13: 243.

Edmundson, A. B., and C. H. W. Hirs. 1961. The amino acid sequence of sperm whale myoglobin. Nature, London, 190: 663.

Ehrenstein, G. v., and F. Lipmann. 1961. Experiments on hemoglobin biosynthesis. Pro. Nat. Acad. Sci. U.S., 47: 941.

Fessas, P. H., and A. Papaspyrou. 1957. New "fast" hemoglobin associated with Thalassemia. Science, 126: 1119.

Fessas, P. H. *et al.* [A. Karaklis and N. Guafakis]. 1961. A further abnormality of foetal haemoglobin. Acta Haematol., 25: 62.

Fincham, J. R. S. 1960. Genetically controlled differences in enzyme activity Advances in Enzymol., 22: 1.

Firschein, L. 1961. Population dynamics of the sickle-cell trait in the Black Caribs of British Honduras, Central America. Am. J. Human Genet., 24: 375.

Garen, A. *et al.* [C. Levinthal and F. Rothman]. 1961. Alterations in alkaline phosphatase induced by mutations. J. chim. phys., 58: 1068.

Garrod, A. E. 1902. The incidence of alkaptonuria, a study in chemical individuality. Lancet, 2: 1616.

Garrod, A. E. 1923. Inborn Errors of Metabolism. Oxford, Oxford University Press.

Gerald, P. S. 1958. The electrophoretic and spectroscopic characterization of Hb M. Blood, 13: 936.

Gerald, P. S. 1960. The Hereditary Methemoglobinemias. *In* The Metabolic Basis of Inherited Disease. (Eds. J. B. Stanbury, J. B. Wyngaarden, D. S. Fredrickson), New York, McGraw Hill Book Co.

Gerald, P. S., and L. K. Diamond. 1958. A new hereditary hemoglobinopathy (the Lepore Trait) and its interaction with Thalassemia trait. Blood, 13: 835.

Gerald, P. S., and M. L. Efron. 1961. Chemical studies of several varieties of Hb M. Pro. Nat. Acad. Sci. U.S., 47: 1758.

Gerald, P. S., and V. M. Ingram. 1961. Recommendations for the nomenclature of hemoglobins. J. Biol. Chem., 236: 2155.

Gerald, P. S. *et al.* [M. Efron and L. K. Diamond]. 1961. Human mutation (the Lepore Hemoglobinopathy) possibly involving two "cistrons". A.M.A. J. Diseases Childhood, 102: 514.

Gluecksohn-Waelsch, S. 1960. The inheritance of hemoglobin types and other biochemical traits in mammals. Symp. on Mammalian Genetics and Reproduction. Oak Ridge National Library, p. 89.

Goldstein, J. *et al.* [G. Guidotti, W. Konigsberg, and R. L. Hill]. 1961. The amino acid sequence around the "reactive sulfhydryl" group of the β chain from human hemoglobin. J. Biol. Chem., 236: PC77.

Gouttas, A. *et al.* [P. H. Fessas, H. Tsevrenis, and E. Xetteri]. 1955. Description d'une nouvelle variété d'anémie hémolytique congénitale. Sang, 26: 911.

Gros, F. *et al.* [H. Hiatt, W. Gilbert, C. G. Kurland, R. W. Risebrough, and J. D. Watson]. 1961. Unstable ribonucleic acid revealed by pulse labeling of *Escherichia coli.* Nature, London, 190: 581.

Guidotti, G. 1960. The action of carboxypeptidase A and B on the separated α and β chains of normal adult human hemoglobin. Biochim. et Biophys. Acta, 42: 177.

Haldane, J. B. S. 1949. Disease and evolution. Ricerca sci. 19, Supplement 68.

Harris, J. I., and V. M. Ingram. 1960. Methods of Sequence Analysis in Proteins. *In* Lab. Manual of Protein Chemistry, Vol. II. (Eds. P. Alexander and R. J. Block), New York, Pergamon.

Havinga, E., and H. A. Itano. 1953. Electrophoretic studies of globins prepared from normal adult and sickle-cell hemoglobins. Pro. Nat. Acad. Sci. U.S., 39: 65.

Helinski, D. R., and C. Yanofsky. 1962. Correspondence between genetic data and the position of amino acid alterations in a protein. Pro. Nat. Acad. Sci. U.S., 48: 173.

Herman, E. C., and C. L. Conley. 1960. Hereditary persistence of fetal hemoglobin. Am. J. Med., 29: 9.

Herrick, J. B. 1910. Peculiar elongated and sickle-cell shaped red blood corpuscles in a case of severe anemia. Arch. internal. Med., 6: 517.

Hill, R. L., and H. C. Schwartz. 1959. A chemical abnormality in hemoglobin G. Nature, London 184: 1903.

Hill, R. L. *et al.* [R. T. Swenson and H. C. Schwartz]. 1960. Characterization of a chemical abnormality in hemoglobin G. J. B. C., 235: 3182.

Hörlein, H., and G. Weber. 1948. Über chronische familiäre Methämoglobinämie und eine neue Modifikation des Methämoglobins. Deut. med. Wochschr., 39: 476.

Horton, B. *et al.* [R. A. Payne, M. T. Bridges, and T. H. J. Huisman]. 1961. studies on an abnormal minor hemoglobin component (Hb–B_2). Clin. Chim. Acta, 6: 246.

Huisman, T. H. J., and J. Drinkwaard. 1955. The N-terminal residues of five different human haemoglobins. Biochim. et Biophys. Acta, 18: 588.

Huisman, T. H. J. *et al.* [K. Punt and J. D. G. Schaad]. 1961. Thalassemia minor associated with Hb–B_2 heterozygosity. A family report. Blood, 17: 747.

Huisman, T. H. J. *et al.* [P. C. van der Schaaf and A. van der Sar]. 1955. Some characteristic properties of hemoglobin C. Blood, 10: 1079.

Hunt, J. A. 1959. Identity of the α chains of adult and foetal human haemoglobins. Nature, London, 183: 1373.

Hunt, J. A., and V. M. Ingram. 1958a. Abnormal human haemoglobins. II. The chymotryptic digestion of the trypsin-resistant "core" of haemoglobin A and S. Biochim. et Biophys. Acta, 28: 546.

Hunt, J. A., and V. M. Ingram. 1958b. Allelomorphism and the chemical differences of the human haemoglobins A, S, and C. Nature, London. 181: 1062.

Hunt, J. A., and V. M. Ingram. 1959. A terminal peptide sequence of human haemoglobin. Nature, London, 184: 640.

Hunt, J. A., and H. Lehmann. 1959. Haemoglobin "Bart's": a foetal haemoglobin without α chains. Nature, London, 184: 872.

Hutton, J. J. *et al.* [J. Bishop, R. Schweet, and E. S. Russell]. 1962. Hemoglobin inheritance in inbred mouse strains. I. Structural differences. Pro. Nat. Acad. Sci. U.S., 48: 1505.

Ingram, V. M. 1957. Gene mutations in human haemoglobin: the chemical difference between normal and sickle-cell haemoglobin. Nature, London, 180: 326.

Ingram, V. M. 1958. Abnormal human haemoglobins. I. The comparison of normal human and sickle-cell haemoglobins by "fingerprinting." Biochim. et Biophys. Acta, 28: 539.

Ingram, V. M. 1959. Abnormal human haemoglobins. III. The chemical difference between normal and sickle-cell haemoglobin. Biochim. et Biophys. Acta, 36: 402.

Ingram, V. M. 1961a. Gene evolution and the haemoglobins. Nature, London, 189: 704.

Ingram, V. M. 1961b. Hemoglobin and its abnormalities. Springfield, Ill., C. C. Thomas.

Ingram, V. M. 1962. A Biochemical Approach to Genetics. *In* Horizons in Biochemistry. (Eds. M. Kasha and B. Pullman), New York, Academic Press, p. 145.

Ingram, V. M., and A. O. W. Stretton. 1959. Genetic basis of the Thalassemia diseases. Nature, London, 184: 1903.

Ingram, V. M., and A. O. W. Stretton. 1961. Human haemoglobin A_2. Nature, London. 190: 1079.

Ingram, V. M., and A. O. W. Stretton. 1962a. Human haemoglobin A_2. I. Comparison of haemoglobins A_2 and A. Biochim. et Biophys. Acta, 62: 456.

Ingram, V. M., and A. O. W. Stretton. 1962b. Human haemoglobin A_2. II. Chemistry of some peptides peculiar to haemoglobin A_2. Biochim. et Biophys. Acta, 63: 20.

Itano, H. A. 1951. A third abnormal hemoglobin associated with hereditary hemolytic anemia. Pro. Nat. Acad. Sci. U.S., 37: 775.

Itano, H. A. 1957. The human hemoglobins: their properties and genetic control. Advances in Protein Chem, 12: 215.

Itano, H. A. 1960. *In* Genetics. New York, Josiah Macy, Jr. Foundation Symp. (Ed. H. E. Sutton), pp. 136–37.

Itano, H. A., and J. V. Neel. 1950. A new inherited abnormality of human hemoglobin. Pro. Nat. Acad. Sci. U.S., 36: 613.

Itano, H. A., and L. Pauling. 1961. Thalassemia and the abnormal human haemoglobins. Nature, London, 191: 398.

Itano, H. A., and E. A. Robinson. 1960. Genetic control of the α and β chains of hemoglobin. Pro. Nat. Acad. Sci. U.S., 46: 1492.

Jacob, F., and J. Monod. 1961. Genetic regulatory mechanisms in the synthesis of proteins. J. Mol. Biol., 3: 318.

Jayle, M. F., and G. Boussier. 1955. Exposés. ann. biochim. méd., 17: 157.

Jones, R. T. *et al.* [W. A. Schroeder, J. E. Balog, and J. R. Vinograd]. 1959. Gross structure of hemoglobin H. J. Am. Chem. Soc., 81: 3161.

Kendrew, J. C. 1961. The three-dimensional structure of a protein molecule. Sci. American, 205: 96.

Kendrew, J. C. *et al.* [R. E. Dickerson, B. E. Strandberg, R. G. Hart, D. R. Davies, D. C. Phillips, and V. C. Shore]. 1960. Structure of myoglobin. A three-dimensional Fourier synthesis at 2 Å resolution. Nature, London, 185: 422.

Kendrew, J. C. *et al.* [H. C. Watson, B. E. Strandberg, R. E. Dickerson, D. C. Phillips, and V. C. Shore]. 1961. The amino acid sequence of sperm whale myoglobin. Nature, London, 190: 666.

Kleihauer, E. *et al.* [H. Braun and K. Betke,]. 1957. Demonstration von Fetalem Hämoglobin in den Erythrocyten eines Blutausstriches. Klin. Wochschr., 35: 637.

Knight, C. A. 1954. Some Recent Developments in the Chemistry of Virus Mutants. *In* Ciba Foundation Symp. (Eds. G. E. W. Wolstenholme and E. C. P. Miller), Boston, Little, Brown & Co., p. 69.

Knopf, P. M. 1962. Ph.D. Thesis: Hemoglobin Synthesis in a Cell-free System, Dept. of Biology, M.I.T., Cambridge, Mass.

Konigsberg, W. *et al.* [G. Guidotti and R. L. Hill]. 1961. The amino acid sequence of the α chain of human hemoglobin. J. Biol. Chem., 236: PC55

Kunkel, H. G., and G. Wallenius. 1955. New hemoglobin in normal adult blood. Science, 122: 288.

Kunkel, H. G. *et al.* [R. Ceppellini, U. Müller-Eberhard, and G. Wolf]. 1957. Observations on the minor basic hemoglobin component in the blood of normal individuals and patients with thalassemia. J. Clin. Invest., 36: 1615.

Lajtha, L. G., and R. Oliver. 1960. Haemopoiesis: Cell Production and its Regulation. *In* Ciba Foundation Symp. (Eds. G. E. W. Wolstenholme and C. M. O'Connor), Boston, Little Brown & Co., p. 289.

Lehmann, H. 1956. Distribution of abnormal haemoglobins. J. Clin. Pathol., 9: 180.

Lehmann, H. 1959. Distribution of Variations in Human Haemoglobin Synthesis. *In* Abnormal Haemoglobins. (Eds. J. H. P. Jonxis and J. F. Delafresnaye), Oxford, Blackwell, p. 202.

Lehmann, H., and J. A. M. Ager. 1960. The hemoglobinopathies and thalassemia. *In* The Metabolic Basis of Inherited Disease. (Eds. J. B. Stanbury, J. B. Wyngaarden, and D. S. Fredrickson), New York, McGraw-Hill.

Lewis, C. B. 1951. Pseudo-allelism and gene evolution. *In* Cold Spring Harbor Symp. on Quant. Biol., 16: 159.

Lie-Injo, L. E. 1961. Haemoglobin "Bart's" and the sickling phenomenon. Nature, London, 191: 1314.

Lie-Injo, L. E., and Lie Hong Gie. 1961. Abnormal haemoglobin production as a probable cause of erythroblastosis and hydrops foetalis in uniovular twins. Acta Haematol., 25: 192.

Low, B., and J. T. Edsall. 1956. Aspects of Protein Structure. *In* Currents in Biochemical Research. (Ed. D. E. Green), New York, Interscience, p. 378.

Marks, P. A. 1960. Discussion. *In* Genetics. New York, Josiah Macy, Jr. Foundation Symp. p. 198.

Marks, P. A. *et al.* [R. T. Gross and J. Banks]. 1961. Evidence for heterogeneity among subjects with glucose-G-P dehydrogenase deficiency. Second Int. Conf. of Human Genetics, Rome, Abstract 136. Publ. Excerpta Medica, Amsterdam.

Marks, P. A. *et al.* [J. Banks and R. T. Gross]. 1962a. Genetic heterogeneity of glucose-6-phosphate dehydrogenase deficiency. Nature, London, 194: 454.

Marks, P. A. *et al.* [C. Wilson, J. Kruh, and F. Gros]. 1962b. Unstable ribonucleic acid in mammalian blood cells. Biochem. Biophys. Res. Comm., 8: 9.

Matthaei, J. H. *et al.* [O. W. Jones, R. G. Martin, and M. W. Nirenberg]. 1962. Characteristics and composition of RNA coding units. Pro. Nat. Acad. Sci. U.S., 48: 666.

McClintock, B. 1956. Controlling elements and the gene. *In* Cold Spring Harbor Symp. on Quant. Biol., 16: 197.

Meyering, C. A. *et al.* [A. C. M. Israels, T. Stebens, and T. H. J. Huisman]. 1959. Studies on the heterogeneity of hemoglobin. Clin. Chim. Acta, 5: 208.

Minnich, V. *et al.* [J. K. Cordonnier, W. J. Williams, and C. V. Moore,]. 1962. α, β and γ hemoglobin peptide chains during the neonatal period with description of a fetal form of Hb D. Blood, 19: 137.

Monod, J., and F. Jacob. 1961. Teleonomic mechanisms in cellular metabolism, growth and differentiation. *In* Cold Spring Harbor Symp. on Quant. Biol., 26: 389.

Moretti, J. *et al.* [G. Boussier and M. F. Jayle]. 1957. Réalisation technique et premières applications de l'électrophorèse sur gel d'amidon. Bull. soc. chim. biol., Paris, 39: 593.

Motulsky, A. G. 1961. The "high fetal hemoglobin" gene: a clue for gene mapping at the human β-hemoglobin locus. Second Int. Conf. Human Genetics, Rome, Abstract 137. Publ. Excerpta Medica, Amsterdam.

Motulsky, A. G. 1962. Controller genes in the synthesis of human haemoglobin. Nature, London 194: 607.

Muller, C. J. 1961. Molecular Evolution. Assen, The Netherlands, Van Gorcum's Medical Library.

Muller, C. J., and S. Kingma. 1961. Haemoglobin Zürich: $\alpha_2^A\beta_2^{63Arg}$. Biochim. et Biophys. Acta, 50: 595.

Murayama, M. 1958. Discussion. *In* Conference on Hemoglobin. Nat. Acad. Sci.-Nat. Research Council, Publ., p. 245.

Murayama, M. 1960. The chemical difference between normal human hemoglobin and Hb I. Federation Proc., 19: 78.

Naughton, M. A., and H. M. Dintzis. 1962. Sequential biosynthesis of the peptide chains of the hemoglobin. Pro. Nat. Acad. Sci. U.S., 48: 1822.

Neeb, H. *et al.* [J. L. Beiboer, J. H. P. Jonxis, J. A. Kaars-Sijpesteijn, and C. J. Muller]. 1961. Homozygous Lepore haemoglobin disease appearing as thalassemia major in two Papuan siblings. Trop. Geograph. Med., 13: 207.

Neel, J. V. 1949. The inheritance of sickle-cell anemia. Science, 110: 64.

Neel, J. V. 1961. The hemoglobin genes: a remarkable example of the clustering of related genetic functions on a single mammalian chromosome. Blood, 18: 769.

Neel, J. V. *et al.* [I. C. Wells and H. A. Itano]. 1951. Familial differences in the proportion of abnormal hemoglobin present in the sickle-cell trait. J. Clin. Invest., 30: 1120.

Parker, W. C., and A. G. Bearn. 1961. Haptoglobin and transferrin variation in humans and primates: two new transferrins in Chinese and Japanese populations. Ann. Human Genetics, 25: 227.

Parker, W. C., and A. G. Bearn. 1962. Studies on the transferrins of adult serum, cord serum, and cerebrospinal fluid. J. Exp Med., 115: 83.

Pauling, L. *et al.* [R. B. Corey and H. R. Branson]. 1951. The structure of proteins: two hydrogen-bonded helical configurations of the polypeptide chain. Pro. Nat. Acad. Sci. U.S., 37: 205.

Pauling, L. *et al.* [H. A. Itano, S. J. Singer, and I. C. Wells]. 1949. Sickle-cell anemia, a molecular disease. Science, 110: 543.

Perutz, M. F. 1962. Relation between structure and sequence of haemoglobin. Nature, London, 194: 914.

Perutz, M. F., and J. M. Mitchison. 1950. State of haemoglobin in sickle-cell anemia. Nature, London, 166: 677.

Perutz, M. F. *et al.* [A. M. Liquori and F. Eirich]. 1951. X-ray and solubility studies of the haemoglobin of sickle-cell anemia patients. Nature, London, 167: 929.

Perutz, M. F. *et al.* [M. G. Rossmann, A. F. Cullis, H. Muirhead, G. Will, and A. T. C. North]. 1960. Structure of haemoglobin. Nature, London, 185: 416.

Ramot, B. *et al.* [A. Szeinberg, Ch. Sheba, A. Adam, and I. Ashkenazi]. 1961. Further investigation on erythrocyte glucose-6-phosphate dehydrogenase deficient subjects: enzyme levels in other tissues and its genetic implications. Second Int. Conf. of Human Genetics, Rome, Abstract 139. Publ. Excerpta Medica, Amsterdam.

Ranney, H. M. 1954. Observations on the inheritance of sickle-cell hemoglobin and hemoglobin C. J. Clin. Invest., 33: 1634.

Ranney, H. M. *et al.* [C. O'Brien and A. S. Jacobs]. 1962. An abnormal human foetal haemoglobin with an abnormal α-polypeptide chain. Nature, London, 194: 743.

Raper, A. B. 1956. Sickling in relation to morbidity from malaria and other diseases. Brit. Med. J., 1: 965.

Raper, A. B. *et al.* [D. B. Gammack, E. R. Huehns, and E. M. Shooter]. 1960. Four hemoglobins in one individual. Brit. Med. J., 2: 1257.

Rich, A. 1952. Studies on the hemoglobin of Cooley's anemia and Cooley's trait. Pro. Nat. Acad. Sci. U.S., 38: 187.

Rigas, D. A. *et al.* [R. D. Koler and E. E. Osgood]. 1955. New hemoglobin possessing a higher electrophoretic mobility than normal adult hemoglobin. Science, 121: 372.

Riggs, A. 1959. Molecular adaptation in haemoglobins: nature of the Bohr effect. Nature, London, 183: 1037.

Riggs, A., and M. Wells. 1961. The oxygen equilibration of sickle-cell haemoglobin. Biochim. et Biophys. Acta, 50: 243.

Roberts, D. F., and A. E. Boyo. 1960. On the stability of haemoglobin gene frequencies in West Africa. Ann. Human Genetics, 24: 375.

Robinson, A. R. *et al.* [M. Robson, A. P. Harrison, and W. W. Zuelzer]. 1957. A new technique for differentiation of hemoglobin. J. Lab. Clin. Med., 50: 745.

Rossi-Fanelli, A. *et al.* [D. Cavallini and C. DeMarco]. 1955. "Amino acid composition of human crystallized myoglobin and haemoglobin. Biochim. et Biophys. Acta, 17: 377.

Rucknagel, D. L., and A. I. Chernoff. 1955. Immunologic studies of haemoglobins. III. Blood, 10: 1092.

Rucknagel, D. L., and J. V. Neel. 1961. The hemoglobinopathies. *In* Progress in Medical Genetics, Vol. I. (Ed. Arthur G. Steinberg), New York, Grune and Stratton.

Schroeder, W. A. 1959. The chemical structure of the normal human hemoglobins. Progr. in Chem. Org. Nat. Prods., 17: 321.

Schroeder, W. A., and G. Matsuda. 1958. N-terminal residues of human fetal hemoglobin. J. Am. Chem Soc., 80: 1521.

Schwartz, H. C. *et al.* [T. H. Spaet, W. W. Zuelzer, J. V. Neel, A. R. Robinson, and S. F. Kaufman]. Combinations of Hb G, Hb S and thalassemia occurring in one family. Blood, 12: 238.

Shooter, E. M. *et al.* [E. R. Skinner, J. P. Garlick, and N. A. Barnicot]. 1960. The electrophoretic characterization of Hb G and a new minor Hb G_2. Brit. J. Haematol., 6: 140.

Siniscalco, M. *et al.* [L. Bernini and B. Latte]. 1961. Linkage data involving G-6-P-D deficiency, colour blindness and hemophilia. Second Int. Conf. of Human Genetics, Rome, Abstract 120. Publ. Excerpta Medica, Amsterdam.

Smith, E. L. 1962. Nucleotide base coding and amino acid replacements in proteins. Pro. Nat. Acad. Sci. U.S., 48: 677.

Smith, E. L. 1962. Nucleotide base coding and amino acid replacements in proteins. II. Pro. Nat. Acad. Sci. U.S., 48: 859.

Smith, E. W., and J. V. Torbert. 1958. Study of two abnormal hemoglobins with evidence for a new genetic locus for hemoglobin formation. Bull. Johns Hopkins Hosp., 102: 38.

Smithies, O. 1959. Zone electrophoresis in starch gels and its application to studies of serum protein. Advances in Protein. Chem., 14: 65.

Smithies, O. 1960. *In* Genetics. New York, Josiah Macy, Jr. Foundation, pp. 129–136.

Smithies, O. *et al.* [G. E. Connell and G. H. Dixon]. 1962. Chromosomal rearrangements and the evolution of haptoglobin genes. Nature, London, 196: 232.

Speyer, J. F. *et al.* [P. Lengyel, C. Basilio, and S. Ochoa]. 1962. Synthetic polynucleotides and the amino acid code. IV. Pro. Nat. Acad. Sci. U.S., 48: 441.

Stein, W. H. *et al.* [H. G. Kunkel, R. D. Cole, D. H. Spackman, and S. Moore]. 1957. Observations on the amino acid composition of human haemoglobins. Biochim. et Biophys. Acta, 24: 640.

Stephens, S. G. 1951. Possible significance of duplication in evolution. Advances in Genet., 4: 247.

Taliaferro, W. H., and J. G. Huck. 1923. The inheritance of sickle-cell anemia in man. Genetics, 8: 594.

Thomas, E. D. *et al.* [H. L. Lochte, Jr., W. B. Greenough, III, and M. Wales]. 1960. In vitro synthesis of foetal and adult haemoglobin by foetal haemotopoietic tissues. Nature, London, 185: 396.

Tsugita, A., and H. Fraenkel-Courat. 1962. The composition of proteins of chemically evoked mutants of TMV RNA. J. Mol. Biol., 4: 73.

Watson, H. C., and J. C. Kendrew. 1961. Comparison between the amino acid sequences of sperm whale myoglobin and of human haemoglobin. Nature, London, 190: 670.

Wells, I. C., and H. A. Itano. 1951. Ratio of sickle-cell anemia hemoglobin to normal hemoglobin in sicklemics. J. Biol. Chem., 188: 65.

Wheeler, J. T., and J. R. Krevans. 1961. Interaction of thalassemia and hereditary persistence of hemoglobin. Clin. Research, 9: 168.

White, J. C., and G. H. Beaven. 1959. Foetal haemoglobin. Brit. Med. Bull., 15: 33.

Wittmann, H. G. 1961. Ansätze zur Entschlüsselung des genetischen Codes. Naturwissenschaften, 48: 729.

Yoshida, A., and T. Tobita. 1960. Studies on the mechanism of protein synthesis. Biochim. et Biophys. Acta, 37: 513.

Zuckerkandl, E. *et al.* [R. T. Jones and L. Pauling]. 1960. A comparison of animal hemoglobins by tryptic peptide pattern analysis. Pro. Nat. Acad. Sci. U.S., 46: 1349.

Zuckerkandl, E., and L. Pauling. 1962. Molecular disease, evolution and genic heterogeneity. *In* Horizons in Biochemistry. (Eds. M. Kasha and B. Pullman), New York, Academic Press, p. 189.

ADDENDA

Edington, G. M., and H. Lehmann. 1955. Expression of the sickle-cell gene in Africa. Brit. Med. J., 2: 1328.

Gratzer, W. B., and A. C. Allison. 1960. Multiple hemoglobins. Biol. Rev., 35: 459.

Harris, J. W. 1950. Studies on the destruction of red blood cells. VIII. Molecular orientation in sickle-cell hemoglobin solutions. Proc. Soc. Exper. Biol. and Med., 75: 197.

INDEX